Game/Set/Match

A Tennis Guide ● Sixth Edition

James E. Bryant

San Jose State University

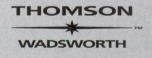

THOMSON

WADSWORTH

Australia • Canada • Mexico • Singapore • Spain
United Kingdom • United States

THOMSON

WADSWORTH

Editor: *April Lemons*
Assistant Editor: *Andrea Kesterke*
Editorial Assistant: *Madinah Chang*
Technology Project Manager: *Travis Metz*
Marketing Manager: *Jennifer Somerville*
Marketing Assistant: *Melanie Wagner*
Advertising Project Manager: *Shemika Britt*
Project Manager: *Kelsey McGee*

Print/Media Buyer: *Karen Hunt*
Permissions Editor: *Elizabeth Zuber*
Production Service and Compositor: *Ash Street Typecrafters, Inc.*
Text and Cover Designer: *Harry Voigt*
Copy Editor: *Carolyn Acheson*
Cover Image: *Ken Reid/Getty Images*
Cover Printing, Printing and Binding: *West Group*

Printed in the United States of America
1 2 3 4 5 6 7 04 03 02 01 00

For more information about our products, contact us at:
Thomson Learning Academic Resource Center
1-800-423-0563
For permission to use material from this text, contact us by:
Phone: 1-800-730-2214
Fax: 1-800-730-2215
Web: http://www.thomsonrights.com

Library of Congress Control Number: 2003100507

ISBN 0-534-57688-5

Wadsworth/Thomson Learning
10 Davis Drive
Belmont, CA 94002-3098
USA

Asia
Thomson Learning
5 Shenton Way #01-01
UIC Building
Singapore 068808

Australia/New Zealand
Thomson Learning
102 Dodds Street
Southbank, Victoria 3006
Australia

Canada
Nelson
1120 Birchmount Road
Toronto, Ontario M1K 5G4
Canada

Europe/Middle East/Africa
Thomson Learning
High Holborn House
50/51 Bedford Row
London WC1R 4LR
United Kingdom

Latin America
Thomson Learning
Seneca, 53
Colonia Polanco
11560 Mexico D.F.
Mexico

Spain/Portugal
Paraninfo
Calle Magallanes, 25
28015 Madrid
Spain

Contents

Preface

This sixth edition of *Game/Set/Match: A Tennis Guide* is written primarily for the beginning or novice player, but it is also appropriate for the intermediate player. It is for students who are actively receiving instruction and planning on continuing to play tennis as a lifelong activity.

The book is written from the perspective of the author as a player and as a college tennis instructor, recognizing that, of the countless ways of playing and teaching the game, the content reflects tennis in a fundamentally sound manner consistent with the majority of those who play and teach the game.

Tennis is a highly popular sport played at all levels of skill and by people of all ages. To be successful requires the development of a foundation of skills, an in-depth comprehension of the intricacy of the flow of the game, and an insight into the rules of play. The game of tennis is played at an intense level of competition by some, and in a spirit of enthusiasm by all who understand that tennis is a game meant to be enjoyed. As played today, tennis is a never-ending learning experience. It is a complex game that, when played and practiced over the years, becomes surprisingly simple, and always remains challenging.

This sixth edition provides players with a visual and written analysis of tennis. Students will profit from reading the descriptions of the skills and reviewing the photographs and diagrams to gain a mental image of how to execute those skills properly. They also will gain from reading and understanding how physical fitness and mental preparation are critical to their improvement and development as players.

Enhanced features in this edition will increase the learning experiences of tennis students. Each chapter has been augmented, particularly from an organizational standpoint. Specifically, all skills and knowledge presented within the text are designed for the beginner. The reality is that students learn at different rates, and university tennis classes are scheduled to cover course content for various periods of time, which means that some beginning material may not be covered in classes that are of shorter duration. Because of that reality, skill-focused chapters have been divided into two parts. At the beginning of any skill-oriented chapter, the most rudimentary skills are presented. Then, at the end of the chapter, more advanced beginning skills are provided. An example of a more advanced beginner skill section would be the slice service as presented in Chapter 4, *Service and Service Return*. The slice serve sometimes is taught as an intermediate serve, but most often actually will be the second serve taught to a beginner. Consequently, chapters that have an advanced skill section like the slice serve are subtitled *Increasing Beginner Skills*.

The 12 chapters in this book could be organized in many different ways. Chapters 1 through 5 are considered the skills chapters and Chapters 6 through 12 are focused on various non-skill aspects of playing. Each of these chapters is designed to enable the student to make sense of the intangibles of tennis. Mental preparation, concepts of strategy, how to practice, how to prepare physically, gaining a concept of tennis ethics and rules, and a general coverage of the intangibles of tennis add to the full coverage of tennis for the beginner. Although all chapters are presented in a logical sequence by the author, it is important to remember that instructors can change the order of the chapters to meet their needs when teaching students.

Adjustments for the sixth edition include updated photographs for each chapter, adding clarity and visualization for the reader and improving clarity and visualization for the student. Self-help sections, *Points to Remember, Common Errors and How to Correct Them,* and *Checkpoints* have been refined and made more consistent. And the 2003 United States Tennis Association's *The Code: The Player's Guide for Unofficiated Matches* has been included in Appendix A.

In sum, this book is a guide for the tennis player who is receiving instruction. I hope everyone who reads and studies this book will continue to grow with the game and reap its rewards through the years.

JEB

Acknowledgments

Ever since 1986 individuals have contributed to the continual development of *Game/Set/Match* as reviewers, models, illustrators, and as sources leading to a book that is as complete and accurate as possible. I want to extend a personal thank you to all who in some way have permitted me to benefit from your knowledge and talents, which has resulted in this book for the beginning tennis player that allows for skill development and growth.

In particular, I want to thank my former students who have given feedback and served as a true test for the practicality and applicability of the book.

Specifically, I want to thank those who have been instrumental in the development of this sixth edition. First, thanks goes to the tennis models: Shane Velez, Kate Hardin, and Robbie Phillips. Without their excellent performance and high skill level the very essence of the visualization of tennis movement would be lost. Second, a thank you to photographer Terrell Lloyd who provided excellent digital photos of tennis as it should be played. The third thank you goes to Oakhurst Country Club Tennis Pro Calvin Thompson, and his assistant Joe Sablan, who provided the Oakhurst (Clayton, California) facilities, scheduling of court time, and names of those who possessed the skills to be the models for the book.

Finally, I thank the reviewers for their comments and ideas: Melanie Mousseau, University of Florida; Stu Schaefer, University of Wisconsin; and Steve VanKanegan, University of Southern California.

James E. Bryant, Ed. D.

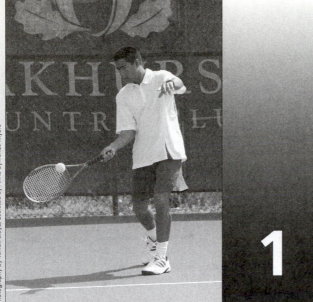

Photography by Terrell Lloyd; assisted by Anna Symonds Myers

1

Preliminaries to the Strokes in Tennis

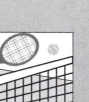

To play tennis, a person has to know how to hold a tennis racket for each stroke, and how to stand and move. Recognizing the spin of the ball, although not of immediate concern to the beginner, is extremely important as the player's skills develop. Additional needs are to comprehend racket-face control and have a feel for the ball as the racket impacts the ball. And learning how to grip and control a tennis racket and how to get ready to hit the ball must be established early in the learning experience.

Basic Tennis Grips

The tennis grip used to hit a given stroke is directly related to execution of that stroke. Selecting a tennis grip that fits the stroke is necessary to complete the stroke using acceptable form.

The *eastern forehand grip*, a universally used grip designed for executing the forehand ground-stroke, is also called the "shake hands" grip (Photos 1.1–1.3). Place your racket hand on the strings of the racket, and bring your hand straight down to the grip. As your hand takes the racket grip, your fingers will be spread along the length of the racket grip with the index finger spread the farthest in a "trigger finger" style, providing control. The thumb will be situated on the back side of the racket, and the thumb and four fingers will form a "V" on the racket grip. The "V" points to the racket shoulder when the player holds the racket in front at a right angle to the body.

The *eastern backhand grip* is a conventional backhand grip used

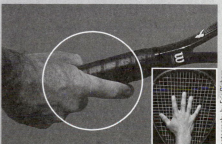

Photo 1.1 "Trigger-finger" position.

Photography by Eric Risberg

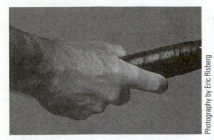

Photo 1.2 Eastern forehand grip (back view).

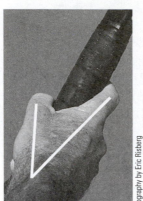

Photo 1.3 Eastern forehand grip (top view).

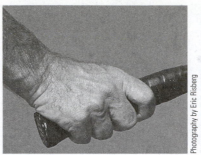

Photo 1.4 Eastern backhand grip (front view).

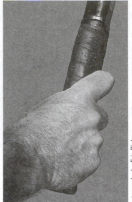

Photo 1.5 Eastern backhand grip (top view).

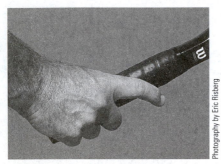

Photo 1.6 Forehand–backhand continental grip (back view).

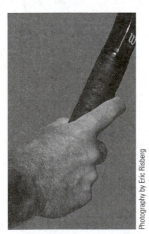

Photo 1.7 Forehand–backhand continental grip (top view).

extensively in tennis (Photos 1.4 and 1.5). From the eastern forehand grip, roll your hand over the top of the racket grip and place your thumb diagonally across the rear plane of the racket grip. From this position you should be able to see all four knuckles of the racket hand when holding the racket perpendicular to the body. When the racket is held in front of the body, the "V" formed by the thumb and fingers will point to the non-racket shoulder.

The *continental forehand grip* and *continental backhand grip* are essentially the same (Photos 1.6 and 1.7). They differ from the eastern forehand and backhand grips in that the hand is placed midway between the positioning of the two eastern grips. The "V" formed by the thumb and fingers points to the middle or center of the body halfway between the racket and non-racket sides of the body when the racket is held in front of the body. The subtle difference between the forehand and the backhand placement of the hand for the continental grip is that, in the forehand grip, the thumb grasps the racket grip, whereas in the backhand the thumb is placed diagonally across the rear of the racket grip.

The *western forehand grip* (Photos 1.8 and 1.9) is often the forehand groundstroke grip of choice by highly skilled players and by developing players who are

taught to impart exaggerated topspin when hitting forehand groundstrokes. This grip also is used by those who pick up a tennis racket for the first time and start to play.

The grip is best achieved by laying the racket on the court and picking it up naturally. The palm of the hand faces flat against and under the back side of the racket grip. The "V" formed by the thumb and fingers, when the racket is held in front of the body, points beyond the racket shoulder.

The *two-hand backhand grip* (Photos 1.10 and 1.11) has become quite popular. It is achieved when the dominant hand grasps the racket grip in a continental grip with the non-dominant hand butted above that grasp in an eastern forehand grip. To execute the stroke, the two-hand backhand grip must be a snug fit of two hands working together. A few players use a two-hand forehand grip, but this grip is not popular and thus is not considered necessary as a choice of grips for the beginning player.

Selecting the grip is based on the stroke used. Eastern forehand grips are used for the forehand groundstroke. The eastern backhand grip is used for the backhand groundstroke and for special serves. The continental grips are used for groundstrokes, net play, and serving. The continental grip has the

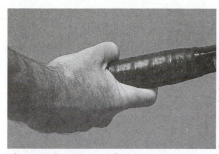

Photo 1.8 Western forehand grip (back view).

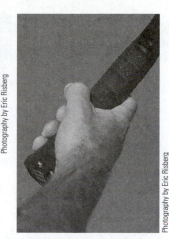

Photo 1.9 Western forehand grip (top view).

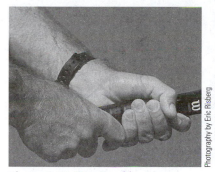

Photo 1.10 Two-hand backhand grip (front view).

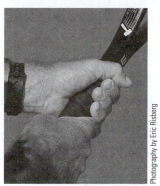

Photo 1.11 Two-hand backhand grip (top view).

added advantage of requiring little in the way of grip adjustment for different strokes; consequently, the strokes are disguised when using this grip. The western forehand is used with success when hitting top-spin forehand groundstrokes.

Players who seek both power and control for their backhand groundstroke often select the two-hand backhand grip. This grip requires the player to cover more distance on a court to reach shots hit wide.

To answer the question of *what grip to use for what stroke*, I suggest that players who intend to stay at the baseline and hit groundstrokes use the eastern grip. An alternative to using the eastern grip when hitting from the baseline is to use a two-hand backhand grip for backhand groundstrokes. When serving, the continental grip will provide control, accuracy, and power for an effective service.

As a beginner, you may want to first use the eastern forehand grip for the serve. As soon as possible, though, you should switch to the continental grip. Going to the net to play a volley shot requires reaction and timing, which means that the grip should not be changed much for a forehand or a backhand volley. The player should maintain a continental grip for play at the net to avoid mis-hitting the ball and being confused at the net.

Points to Remember

Grip

1. Keep the fingers spread down the racket grip with the index finger serving as a "trigger finger."

2. Be aware of the location of the "V" in relation to the racket and non-racket shoulders.

3. Grasp the racket firmly when assuming a grip.

4. Understand the subtle differences between each grip and the purpose for each.

Common Errors and How to Correct Them (Grip)

The Error	What Causes the Error	To Correct the Error
Lack of control of the racket.	Grasping the racket in a fist-like position.	Make sure the fingers are spread along the racket grip with a trigger finger.
Mis-hitting a ball or poor execution.	Grip is too tight.	Relax the grip. Grasp the racket firmly, not tightly.
	Grip is too loose.	Tighten the grip. Grasp the racket firmly, not tightly. Check grip size. If the grip is too small, the racket will turn in the hand when a return shot has high velocity.
	Wrong grip for the stroke.	Check purpose for each grip.

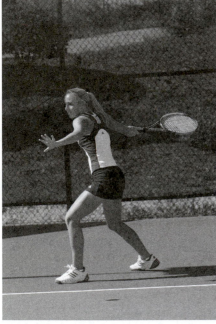

Photo 1.12 Forehand groundstroke follow-through.

Photo 1.13 Backhand groundstroke.

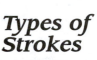

Types of Strokes

As an introduction to strokes in tennis, a definition of the various strokes should enable better understanding of the basic skills of the game. **Groundstrokes** are either forehand or backhand.

The basic *forehand groundstroke* (Photo 1.12) is hit from the baseline following the bounce of the ball. The stroke is executed with a swinging action that produces a flat, no-spin (actually, most flat shots have a small amount of topspin) movement to the ball.

The *backhand groundstroke* (Photo 1.13) is played under the same conditions as the forehand groundstroke, with the same ball action. Both are swinging action strokes with the forehand hit on the racket side of the body and the backhand hit on the non-racket side of the body.

Both strokes are foundations for more advanced strokes, including *topspin* and *slice (underspin) groundstrokes.* These **approach shots**, which are an extension of

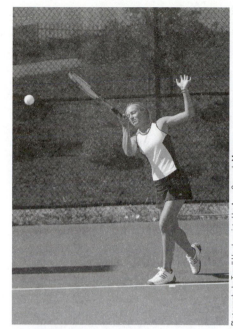

Photography by Terrell Lloyd; assisted by Anna Symonds Myers

Photo 1.14 Lob.

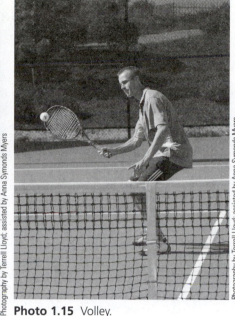

Photography by Terrell Lloyd; assisted by Anna Symonds Myers

Photo 1.15 Volley.

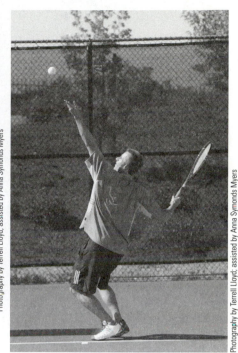

Photography by Terrell Lloyd; assisted by Anna Symonds Myers

Photo 1.16 Flat serve.

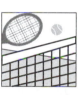

Photography by Terrell Lloyd; assisted by Anna Symonds Myers

Photo 1.17 Overhead.

groundstrokes, are characterized by a player advancing to the middle of the court to hit a ball. All **lobs** (Photo 1.14) are also an extension of groundstrokes in terms of the swinging action; they have a lifting action designed to hit the ball deep to the baseline and with a loft.

The **volley** (Photo 1.15) is a punching action characterized by playing the ball before it contacts the court surface. Both forehand and backhand volleys usually are played at the net. The **half-volley** is an extension of a volley shot.

The fourth type of stroke is the basic **flat serve** (Photo 1.16), and it is described as a throwing action. Strokes that develop from the flat service are the slice service (sidespin), the topspin service, and an advanced stroke known as the American twist (another sidespin rotation).

The **overhead** (Photo 1.17) is a continuation of the basic flat service. Key parts of the serve are reflected in the overhead stroke. It differs from the serve in that the ball is hit either on the fly or after a bounce on the court surface when the offensive player is positioned near the net.

Feel and Timing of the Tennis Ball

Developing a **feel** for the tennis ball is a prerequisite for successful tennis play. Regardless of racket control, spin of the ball, and various stroke fundamentals, execution of each stroke depends on feeling for the ball through *eye–hand coordination*, *timing*, and *focus*.

Eye–hand coordination is based on past experiences of throwing and catching an object similar in size to a tennis ball. The swinging, throwing, and punching actions associated with tennis are fundamental to the ball games of batting, throwing, and catching that most American children play during their childhood. If you have played softball or racquetball or have engaged in activities such as playing catch, the game of tennis will be easy for you compared to individuals who have not had those experiences.

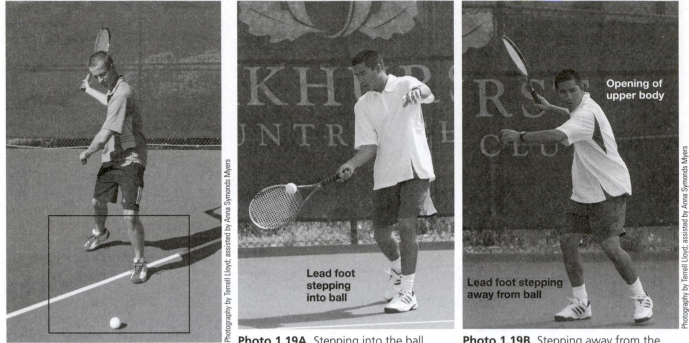

Photo 1.18 Position of ball and feet away and behind the ball.

Photo 1.19A Stepping into the ball.

Photo 1.19B Stepping away from the ball.

Timing in tennis is related to where the ball eventually will be positioned to be hit rather than where it bounced originally. You must comprehend where the ball will go after it bounces, and set up behind and away from the ball so you can step into the ball to hit it (Photo 1.18). Players tend to get too close to the ball, or too far away, which causes them to lurch to hit the ball rather than step smoothly into the ball. If the ball is too far away, the player can adjust (and not lose timing) by stepping toward the ball with a weight transfer (Photo 1.19A). If the ball is too close, the player should step away, yet forward, to hit the ball (Photo 1.19B). The key factor in stepping away is to open the upper body as the racket is brought through the ball at contact.

Part of timing involves controlling the speed of the racket head. Players under pressure tend to swing too hard or too fast, particularly with return of service. You must remember to play from a relaxed position and control the racket-head speed. The same is true with hitting overhead smashes and groundstrokes when the opposing player is at the net. The added pressure tends to break down timing, forcing the player to rush through the stroke. The focal points have to be *relaxation*, *confidence* in hitting the ball, and *concentration* on the ball. Timing is improved immeasurably by watching the ball as long as possible. This is the part of focus that is most often ignored.

The ability to **focus** is extremely important in tennis. The ability to "see" the ball and perceive the racket striking the ball will help the developing player improve rapidly. Being able to focus on the ball is based on the same past experiences as with eye–hand coordination. Focus requires recognizing the bounce of the ball in terms of height, estimating distance of the ball from the player, and judging the relationship of the

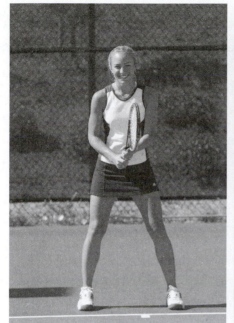

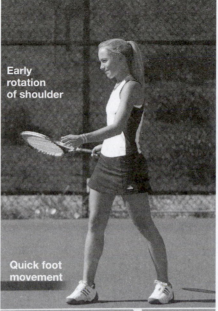

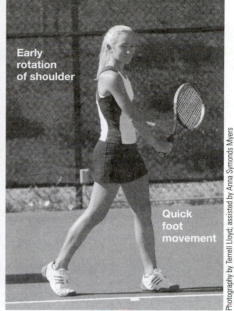

Photo 1.20A Ready position for a groundstroke.

Photo 1.20B Ready position—turn of shoulders (forehand).

Photo 1.20C Ready position—turn of shoulders (backhand).

Photography by Terrell Lloyd; assisted by Anna Symonds Myers

ball to the body. In addition, focus entails moving to the ball, transferring the weight into the ball at contact, and being in the correct position at the correct time. A final consideration in focusing is the ability to block all outside distractions and keep the tennis ball as the only target.

The foundation for timing and feel for the ball rests with establishing a **ready position** from which to hit groundstrokes and volleys (Photo 1.20A). The ready position is the first actual skill presented for the developing player, and it is the foundation for all strokes.

The feet should be spaced slightly wider than shoulder-width and parallel to each other. The knees are slightly bent, and the weight of the body is centered over the balls of the feet. The buttocks should be "down," with the upper body leaning slightly forward in a straight alignment. The head should be "up," looking toward the ball on

the opposite side of the net. The racket is held "up" with a forehand grip on the handle, with the non-racket hand lightly touching the throat of the racket. The racket head is above the hands, and the elbows are clear of the body.

The ready position gives the player the opportunity to move equally to the right or left, as well as to advance forward or retreat backward. The first response from a player in the ready position is to rotate the shoulders immediately when recognizing the direction of the ball from across the net (Photos 1.20B and 1.20C). A player with good mobility will be able to move the feet quickly from the ready position. If a player can be relaxed in a ready position, keep the weight on the balls of the feet, and then react to the approaching ball with an early turn of the shoulders and quick foot movement, the stroke has been initiated positively.

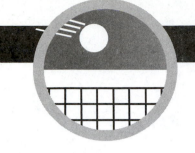

Points to Remember

Ready Position

1. Maintain a base with the feet shoulder-width apart.
2. Focus on the ball on the other side of the net.
3. Keep the knees bent slightly and the weight on the balls of the feet.
4. Be relaxed and ready to react.
5. As the ball crosses the net, turn the shoulders and move the feet.

Common Errors and How to Correct Them (Ready Position)

The Error	What Causes the Error	To Correct the Error
Falling off balance.	Feet too close together.	Widen the base.
Incorrect timing of the ball.	Not focusing on the ball and not getting the shoulders rotated early with the feet moving.	Watch the seams of the ball and rotate your shoulders early.

Increasing Beginner Skills: Racket Control and Ball Spin

Your first concern as a beginning player is to simply hit the ball when it comes to you. As your skills improve, you will have to direct attention to racket control and ball spin to improve further.

Racket control is essential to good strokes, and thus to successful play. When swinging a racket, three basic actions will provide racket-head control and consequently will accomplish a stroke. The basic **swinging action** is reflected in the forehand and backhand ground-strokes and the various lobs. The serve and overhead strokes are described through the *action of throwing*. The *punch action* is used with forehand and backhand volleys. By executing each of these actions or patterns, you will eliminate all extraneous motion, which will help you to simplify the action of each stroke.

Also, three basic **racket face** positions will affect the control and flight pattern of the ball and the bounce of the ball on the surface of the court. The effect of these three positions on the resulting action of the ball depends on the speed of the racket head while hitting through the ball and on the angle of the racket face when it contacts the ball. If contact is made with the *racket face flat* to the ball (Photo 1.21), the flight of the ball will be straight, and the ball will fall to the

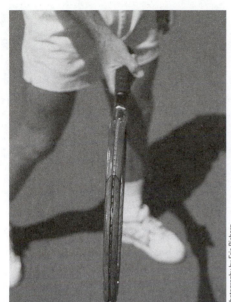

Photo 1.21 Flat racket face.

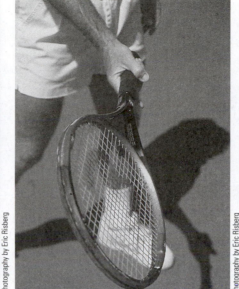

Photo 1.22 Open racket face.

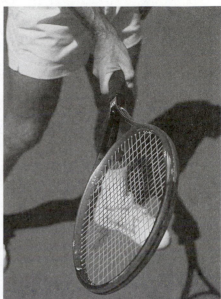

Photo 1.23 Closed racket face.

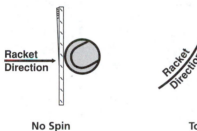

No Spin

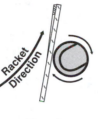

Topspin

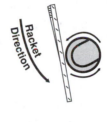

Underspin

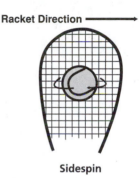

Sidespin

Figure 1.1   Basic actions for balls in flight.

court surface due to gravity. An **open racket face** (Photo 1.22) will cause the ball to have a floating action in its flight, spinning in a backward motion. A *closed racket face* (Photo 1.23) will force the flight pattern of the ball downward because the ball has a forward spin.

Each racket face position is important to all skill levels. Understanding what causes the drop or rise of the ball gives the beginning player greater insight into the total concept of hitting the ball and reacting to the bounce.

Comprehending spins is a direct carryover from understanding racket head and racket face control. A tennis shot that is hit without spin is affected by three aspects of the overall stroke.

1. As the ball strikes the racket face, a direct force is applied to the ball, which provides velocity and determines the ball's flight pattern.

2. That velocity is countered by air resistance and gravity; the former impedes the velocity of the tennis ball and the latter pulls the ball down toward the court.

3. The ball will strike the tennis court surface at an angle equal to the rebound of the ball off the court surface.

When a ball spins in its flight pattern, the tennis player also must cope with the behavior of the ball as it strikes the court surface. There are three *basic spinning actions for balls in flight* (see Figure 1.1).

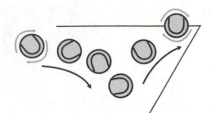

Action of ball striking court—topspin

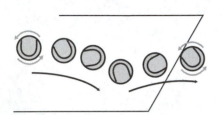

Action of ball striking court—underspin

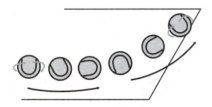

Action of ball striking court—sidespin

Figure 1.2 Basic actions for ball striking the court.

1. **Topspin** is caused by the action of the top surface of the ball rotating against air resistance. This creates friction on the top part of the ball, forcing the ball in a downward path.

2. **Underspin** is caused by the bottom of the ball meeting air resistance and forcing the ball to stay up longer than normally is found with a non-spinning ball.

3. **Sidespin** is created when the side of the ball meets air resistance and pressure. This causes the ball to veer to the opposite side.

The *action of the ball striking the court surface* is the end result of racket control action on the ball and the spin of the flight of the ball (Figure 1.2). As the tennis ball makes contact with the tennis court, the ball will behave in a highly predictable manner. A *topspin* action will hit the court surface with a high, deep bounce because of the forward rotation of the ball. A ball hit with *underspin* usually is hit with power and at a low angle, creating a skidding action as ball meets surface. The *sidespin* strikes the court with the same action and direction as the sidespin on the ball.

In summary, racket control and spin of the ball have a cause–effect relationship. A flat racket face at contact will cause a flat flight pattern and a flat equal-angle bounce off the court. An open racket face will result in underspin during the flight of the ball and a skidding action upon contact with the court surface. A closed racket face will provide a topspin ball action with a resulting high and deep bounce off the court surface. The player should understand that these two racket positions for the slice and topspin groundstrokes produce only a subtle change at contact.

A closed racket face striking the ball on the side will create a sidespin action followed by a sideward bounce when the ball strikes the court. The beginning player has to understand the various spins applied to a ball in order to cope with balls hit with spin and to learn how to supply spin to various strokes.

Checkpoints ✔✔

1. The eastern forehand grip is described as
   a. trigger finger, V formed by index finger and thumb with V pointed to racket shoulder.
   b. grasp of racket, V formed by index finger and thumb with V pointed to the racket shoulder.
   c. trigger finger, V formed by index finger and thumb with V pointed to center of chest.
   d. trigger finger, V formed by index finger and thumb with V pointed to non-racket shoulder.

2. The continental grip is described as
   a. similar to a two-handed grip.
   b. halfway between an eastern forehand and western forehand grip.
   c. halfway between an eastern forehand and eastern backhand grip.
   d. halfway between an eastern backhand and western forehand grip.

3. The continental grip is used most effectively for
   a. playing the baseline.
   b. playing the baseline and the net.
   c. playing the baseline and serve.
   d. playing the net and serve.

4. The basic racket control actions are
   a. punch action, swing action, and throw action.
   b. punch action and swing action.
   c. throw action and swing action.
   d. punch action and throw action.

5. The three types of spin imparted on a ball in flight are
   a. topspin, sidespin, underspin.
   b. reverse spin, topspin, backspin.
   c. reverse spin, sidespin, topspin.
   d. sidespin, reverse spin, slice.

6. Feel for the tennis ball requires
   a. eye-hand coordination, focus, and foot coordination.
   b. eye-hand coordination, timing, and focus.
   c. focus, foot coordination, and timing.
   d. foot coordination, eye-hand coordination, and timing.

7. The first response from a ready position is to
   a. rotate the shoulders.
   b. turn the racket-side shoulder.
   c. turn the non-racket-side shoulder.
   d. rotate the shoulders with the direction of the ball seen across the net.

8. The tennis racket should be grasped
   a. tightly.
   b. loosely.
   c. firmly.
   d. in a fist-like grip.

Answers to Checkpoints can be found on page 147.

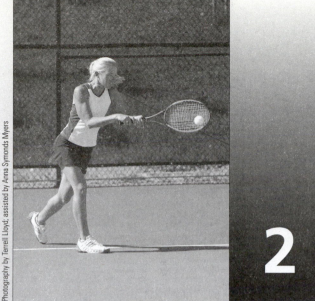

Photography by Terrell Lloyd; assisted by Anna Symonds Myers

2

Groundstrokes

Groundstrokes are crucial to success in tennis. They are executed by the player hitting the tennis ball from the baseline area following one bounce of the ball on the court. The **groundstroke** involves a swinging action designed to hit the ball deep to the opponent's baseline. Both the **forehand** and the **backhand** groundstrokes develop from the basic (little spin) flat stroke and evolve into other groundstrokes termed **topspin** and **slice** (underspin) groundstrokes. To initiate the groundstroke, get in the ready position and then decide whether to use the forehand or the backhand.

Groundstrokes— Basic Forehand

The *basic forehand groundstroke* is the foundation for all forehands hit with spin. It is the stroke players use most often if they are given the choice between a backhand and a forehand.

The eastern forehand grip—also known as the "shake hands" grip—is used to execute the basic forehand groundstroke. The basic forehand groundstroke has three stages: preparing to hit the ball, contacting the ball, and following through. Each stage must be performed in sequence.

Preparing To Hit the Ball

When preparing to hit the ball, the player is in the ready position. Two reactions follow:

1. Rotation of the shoulders.

2. Movement of the feet. As a result of the shoulder and foot movement, the racket is placed in an early backswing position. To do this, the player may either bring the racket straight back or loop the racket. Either is acceptable because the goal is to get the racket back in a low position to hit from a semi-low to a high position. The loop is emphasized as an example in this situation.

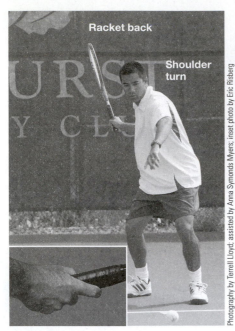

Racket back

Shoulder turn

Photography by Terrell Lloyd; assisted by Anna Symonds Myers; inset photo by Eric Risberg

Photo 2.1 Pull the racket back in a line even with the eye (eastern forehand grip).

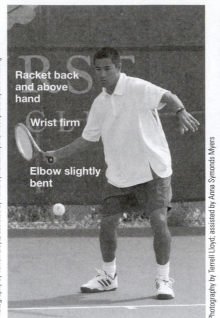

Racket back and above hand

Wrist firm

Elbow slightly bent

Photography by Terrell Lloyd; assisted by Anna Symonds Myers

Photo 2.2 Backswing—racket perpendicular and high.

Racket slightly below hand

Transfer weight forward

Lead leg bent

Photography by Terrell Lloyd; assisted by Anna Symonds Myers

Photo 2.3 Preparation for contact with the ball.

The **loop** is divided into three parts:

1. The shoulders turn, allowing the racket to pull back in a line even with the eye (Photo 2.1).

2. The racket moves to a general perpendicular position aligned to the fence located behind the baseline, with the racket positioned slightly higher than the hand and wrist (Photo 2.2).

3. The racket drops below the line of the flight of the ball at about a 12-inch position below and behind the intended contact area to the ball (Photo 2.3). The loop will provide rhythm to the swing, add extra velocity to the ball following impact, and ensure a grooved swing.

The full pattern for this preparation is to bring the racket back as quickly as possible by reacting early to the ball and turning the shoulders at a 45-degree angle to begin inertia. As the racket starts back in the loop following the shoulder turn, both feet will move and pivot automatically to accommodate the upper

body turn. When the racket moves to a position perpendicular to the fence beyond the back court, the wrist and arm should be firm, with the elbow bent slightly and away from the body. The final part of the preparation is to bend the legs.

Contact with the Ball

Contact with the ball begins when the racket moves from the backswing in a semi-low to a high pattern. The weight is transferred from back foot to lead foot. The lead leg is bent at contact while the back leg is beginning to straighten. The palm of the hand grasping the racket is behind the ball at impact, with a firm wrist and with the arm extended 8 to 10 inches from the body. The non-racket arm is extended toward the ball, giving direction to the ball and balance to the body.

The ball is hit off the lead leg at slightly above mid-thigh to above waist level. The sequence of backswing to contact with the ball requires stepping into the ball, transferring the weight forward, and keeping the ball away from the body at a position toward the net and sideline (Photo 2.3).

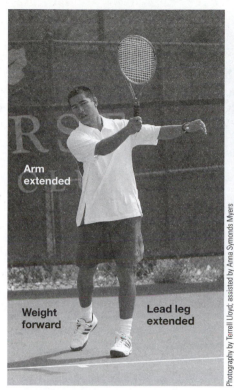

Arm extended

Weight forward

Lead leg extended

Photography by Terrell Lloyd; assisted by Anna Symonds Myers

Photo 2.4 Forehand groundstroke follow-through.

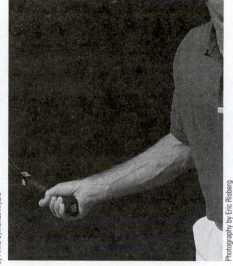

Photography by Eric Risberg

Photo 2.5 Forehand groundstroke closeup of shoulder, elbow, and wrist.

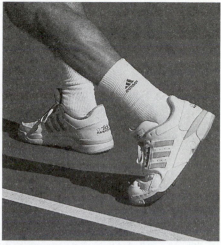

Photography by Eric Risberg

Photo 2.6 Weight centered over balls of the feet.

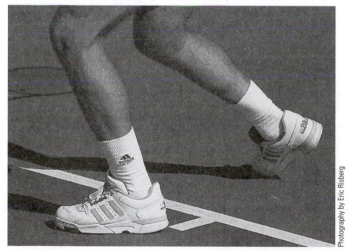

Photography by Eric Risberg

Photo 2.7 Pivoting and lifting actions through the stroke.

Follow Through

The final part of the sequence is the *follow-through*. The wrist remains firm and fixed and the arm extends out across the body, with the inside of the upper arm touching the chin. The legs lift throughout the follow-through, with the lead leg fully extended and the back leg slightly bent. The purpose of the follow through is to eliminate premature lifting or pulling of the ball before it leaves the racket strings at contact (Photo 2.4).

Crucial to executing the stroke are the *position of the elbow and wrist* and the *transfer of weight*. The wrist and arm *must* remain firm but relaxed throughout the stroke. The tendency is to lay back the wrist and to hyperextend the elbow. The wrist should not rotate, and the elbow should remain slightly bent. Both should remain firm (Photo 2.5).

Weight transfer provides the needed drive behind the ball, with the center of gravity directed forward through the stroke by a stepping motion into the ball. During the weight transfer, the legs must be bent with a change in the degree of bend through the full stroke.

Footwork and *early preparation* are both critical to success with the forehand groundstroke. Footwork supplies the mobility and balance that provide the base for the stroke, and it sets the stage for weight transfer and leg power. Weight has to be centered over the balls of the feet to effect ease of movement, and the pivoting and lifting actions aid throughout the stroke in placing the body in a position to hit the ball (Photos 2.6 and 2.7). The early preparation includes good shoulder

Basic Forehand Groundstroke

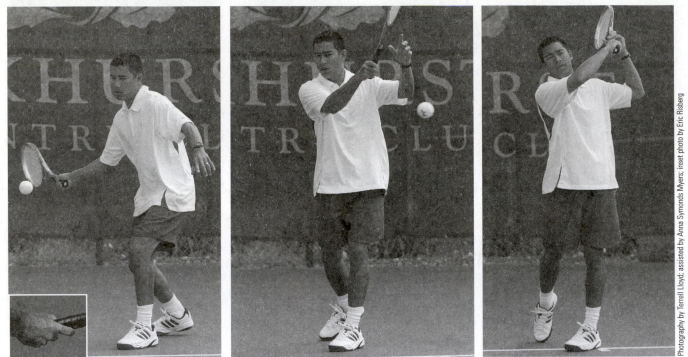

Photo 2.8A Backswing.   **Photo 2.8B** Contact.   **Photo 2.8C** Follow-through.

rotation and accompanying foot pivot with a loop backswing. That early response to the opponent's shot is the base for all that follows.

The stroke must be performed in full sequence, with a fluid movement from one part to the next. Any jerky, non-grooved action will detract from the stroke. The acceptable sequence has to include coordination of feet, legs, shoulder, arm, and wrist (Photos 2.8A–C).

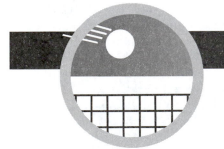

Points to Remember

Basic Forehand Groundstroke

1. Always start from a ready position.
2. Prepare with an early shoulder rotation and pivot of the feet.
3. Activate the loop or a straight-back backswing.
4. Step into the ball at contact by transferring your weight forward.
5. Contact the ball with the palm-of-the-hand position and firm wrist.
6. Swing from slightly low to high, with the follow-through extending high and across the body.
7. Maintain a full, synchronized sequence to the timing of the stroke.

Common Errors and How to Correct Them
(Basic Forehand Groundstroke)

The Error	What Causes the Error	To Correct the Error
Ball pulled to the non-racket side of the court.	Hitting too far out in front of the body or turning the racket shoulder too much through the stroke.	Step into the ball, hitting off the lead leg. Keep your non-racket shoulder consistent with transfer of weight forward. Keep your non-racket hand out in front of your body.
Ball directed to the near racket side of the court.	Being late in the backswing position, backswing beyond the perpendicular position to the fence, or laying the wrist too far back.	React early to the flight of the ball with a 45-degree turn of the shoulders, initiating an early backswing.
Balls hit short with little velocity.	Not stepping into the ball with weight transfer, and poor racket pattern from high to slightly low. Racket also may be too high at the lowest part of the backswing.	Transfer your weight into the ball at contact. Change the swinging pattern to slightly low to high.
Balls hit long or high against opponent's back fence.	Hitting the ball with poor timing, or too hard with the weight on the back foot, or in a lifting pattern at contact; also "breaking wrist" at contact.	Synchronize the timing of the stroke with the slightly low-to-high racket pattern; use good weight transfer. Keep your wrist firm; don't lean back at contact with the ball.

Groundstrokes—Basic Backhand

The basic backhand groundstroke is the easier of the two strokes (forehand vs. backhand) to hit mechanically, yet it is the stroke that most players fail to execute successfully in competition. Hitting a backhand is easy and fun, but first the player must develop confidence.

The *grip* still used for the basic backhand is the *eastern backhand grip*, with the hand rolled onto the top of the racket grip so the "V" is pointed to the non-racket shoulder when the racket is held in front of the body. Another guide for the grip is to align the knuckles of the racket hand with the net when the racket makes contact with the ball.

As with all forehand strokes and backhands, the stroke has three phases that all mesh into a consistent, grooved feeling. *Preparation in hitting the ball* is based on an early reaction to the ball with an immediate rotation of both shoulders. The feet pivot during the shoulder rotation, and the racket starts its backswing movement with either the loop or straight back technique. The loop is pulled back at eye level and then dropped about 8 inches below the contact point of the ball (Photo 2.9).

A change of grips also occurs in the preparation phase. The player begins the stroke from a ready position with an eastern forehand grip.

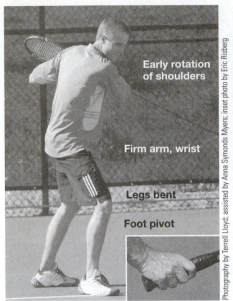

Early rotation of shoulders

Firm arm, wrist

Legs bent

Foot pivot

Photo 2.9 Backhand groundstroke preparation (eastern backhand grip).

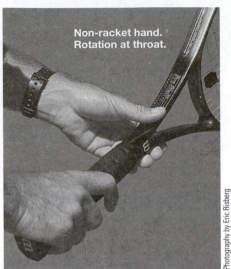

Non-racket hand. Rotation at throat.

Photo 2.10 Changing grips for the backhand.

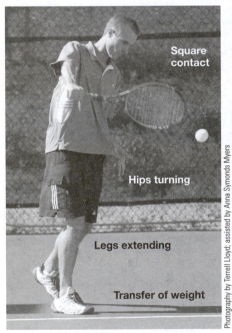

Square contact

Hips turning

Legs extending

Transfer of weight

Photo 2.11 Backhand groundstroke contact.

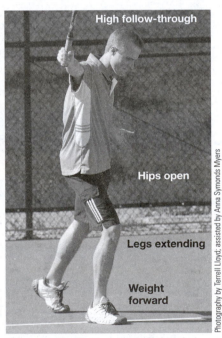

High follow-through

Hips open

Legs extending

Weight forward

Photo 2.12 Backhand groundstroke follow-through.

As the player reacts to the ball and turns the shoulders and pivots the feet, the racket begins its backward journey. As the racket moves back, the player uses the non-racket hand to adjust the grip by turning the racket at the throat until the top of the hand is seen as the racket follows the shoulder to the backswing position (Photo 2.10).

The non-racket hand stays in contact with the throat of the racket throughout the backswing and into the movement forward to hit the ball. During the final extension backward the racket is perpendicular to the back fence. The weight of the body is centered over the back foot and the legs are bent, permitting the body to be coiled for the next phase of the stroke.

Contact with the ball occurs with a semi-low-to-high swinging pattern that will ensure direction for the ball. The shoulder leads the elbow into the swing, and the elbow leads the wrist. This provides an accumulating effect so at contact the racket is square to the ball and the joint alignment from shoulder to wrist is a straight line. That joint alignment provides a firm base of support as the ball strikes the racket face. The weight of the body is transferred to the lead leg just prior to contact with the ball, and the position of the racket to the lead leg at contact is mid-thigh to above waist level (Photo 2.11).

The *follow-through* is an extension of the semi-low-to-high swinging action, with the weight continuing forward off the lead leg as the lead leg straightens and the back leg bends slightly (Photo 2.12). This provides a degree of balance to the base of the stroke. The wrist remains firm as the racket finishes high, facing the racket side of the sideline.

Key elements in the basic backhand groundstroke are the *wrist, elbow,* and *shoulder positions.* The initial shoulder turn followed by the shoulder leading into the stroke are essential movements in completing the action. The elbow and the wrist never should be physically ahead of the racket (Photo 2.13). The racket should rotate around the wrist, and the wrist should rotate around the elbow from backswing to contact with the ball.

At follow-through the racket should lead the wrist and elbow. If the elbow or wrist leads the racket

Photography by Terrell Lloyd; assisted by Anna Symonds Myers; inset photo by Eric Risberg

Photography by Eric Risberg

Photography by Terrell Lloyd; assisted by Anna Symonds Myers

Photography by Terrell Lloyd; assisted by Anna Symonds Myers

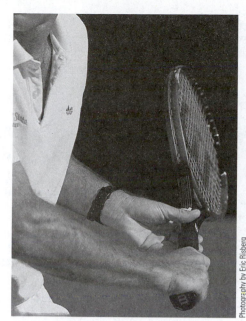

Photo 2.13 Backhand groundstroke closeup of shoulder, elbow, and wrist.

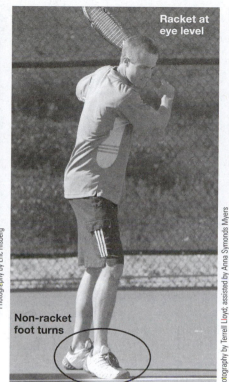

Photo 2.14 Backhand groundstroke loop—pull the racket back at eye level.

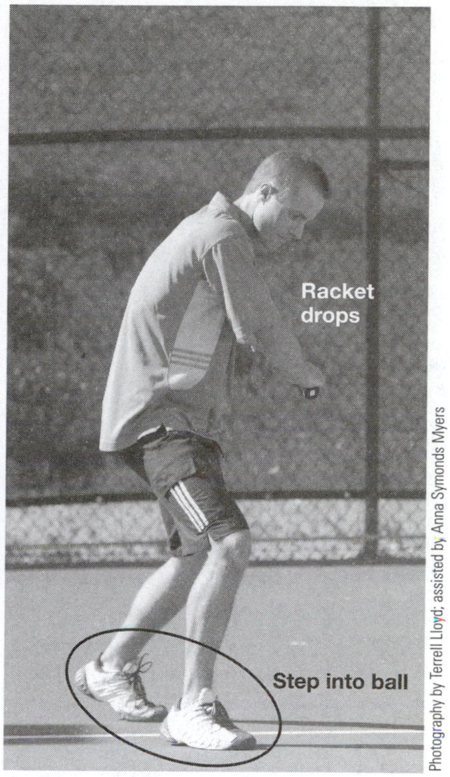

Photo 2.15 Backhand groundstroke loop—drop the racket below the projected contact point of the ball.

at contact, a pushing action will result, decreasing the velocity of the ball. The racket arm stays closer to the body—at a distance of perhaps 6 to 8 inches—than with the forehand.

Racket control, weight transfer, footwork, and *leg power* all contribute to the success or failure of the backhand groundstroke. Racket control is characterized by the loop—pulling the racket back at eye level (Photo 2.14), then dropping the racket below the projected contact point of the ball (Photo 2.15).

Balance and weight transfer occur when the player uses proper footwork from the ready position to the final follow-through. The critical part of the footwork involves the singular turn of the non-racket foot when the shoulder rotates (Photo 2.14—see circle) and the subsequent stepping into the ball with the racket-side foot just prior to contact with

the ball (Photo 2.15—see circle). The weight transfer is a total exchange from moving weight from the back foot during preparation to the lead leg at contact on through follow-through.

The full sequence of actions involved in the basic backhand groundstroke will determine the outcome of the stroke. Movement must be a fluid sequence void of all jerky or shaky movement. That sequence should include coordination of shoulders, feet, legs, elbow, and wrist into a mechanically smooth, grooved stroke that causes the racket to contact the ball in a nearly square position and that flows to an ultimate follow-through (Photos 2.16A–C). As a final thought, the mechanics of the stroke have to be combined with the belief that the backhand is easier to execute and mechanically more sound than the forehand.

Basic Backhand Groundstroke

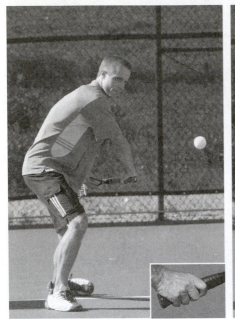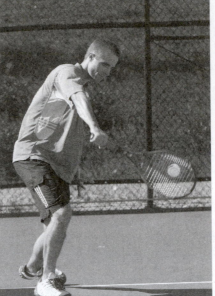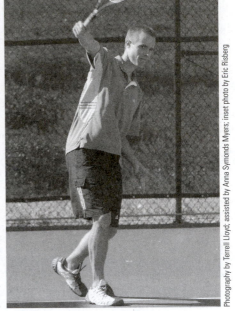

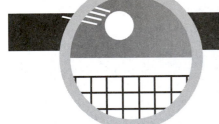

Photo 2.16A Backswing.   **Photo 2.16B** Contact.   **Photo 2.16C** Follow-through.

Photography by Terrell Lloyd; assisted by Anna Symonds Myers; inset photo by Eric Risberg

Points to Remember

Basic Backhand Groundstroke

1. Always start from the ready position.
2. Prepare with an early shoulder rotation and pivot of the feet.
3. Activate the loop or a straight-back motion backswing.
4. Change the grip from eastern forehand to eastern backhand as the racket is brought to the backswing position.
5. Keep a firm wrist, and keep the elbow and wrist behind the racket to contact.
6. Transfer the weight from the back to the front foot as the racket moves from backswing to contact to follow-through.
7. Swing low to high, with the racket finishing high and parallel to the racket-side sideline.
8. Keep a full synchronized sequence to the timing of the stroke.

Common Errors and How to Correct Them
(Basic Backhand Groundstroke)

The Error	What Causes the Error	To Correct the Error
Ball pulled to the non-racket side of the court.	Hitting too far out in front of the body, or turning the racket shoulder too early.	Stay sideways as long as you can during the swing.
Ball directed to the non-racket side of the court.	Too late in shoulder turn to initiate a backswing.	Anticipate early and turn your shoulder to set up the backswing.
Ball hit short or into the net with little velocity.	Not stepping into the ball at contact with minimal weight transfer, or not keeping your racket arm or elbow extended or fixed through contact.	Step into the ball and transfer your weight forward. Hit with a flat racket face and follow a racket pattern from semi-low to high. Hit with an extended and fixed racket arm.
Ball hit long or high against opponent's fence.	Hitting with poor timing, or weight, on back foot. Also opening racket face too much and not following through, or the racket side elbow may be raised.	Synchronize the timing and transfer your weight to the lead foot at contact and follow-through. Step into the ball at contact. Make sure to follow through. Also check your grip and make sure it is an eastern backhand grip.

Groundstrokes—Two-hand Backhand

The two-hand backhand is immensely popular today with people who need the added strength for force and velocity, as well as more control, particularly the beginner who has trouble hitting the **sweet spot** of the racket face. The player using the two-hand backhand will gain confidence in the backhand, but at the same time sacrifice the reach related to the conventional backhand stroke. With the exception of the lack of reach, the two-hand backhand provides the opportunity to hit both topspin and slice without changing grips; rather, the change occurs in swing action and in the position of the arms in reference to the body.

In the *two-hand backhand*, the dominant hand grips the racket with a continental grip at the butt end of the racket handle. The non-dominant hand rests on top of the racket-side hand in an eastern forehand grip. The heel of the support hand is nestled snugly between the thumb and index finger of the racket-side hand.

Preparation for hitting the ball involves basic rotation of the shoulders, except that the rotation will be limited because of the two-hand position. Rather than a loop backswing, the racket is brought straight back and then dropped low toward the feet. The same foot pivot and weight transfer occur with the two-hand backhand as with the conventional eastern forehand and backhand (Photo 2.17A).

Contact with the ball involves continuation of the low-to-high pattern with the arms close to the body

Basic Two-Hand Backhand Groundstroke

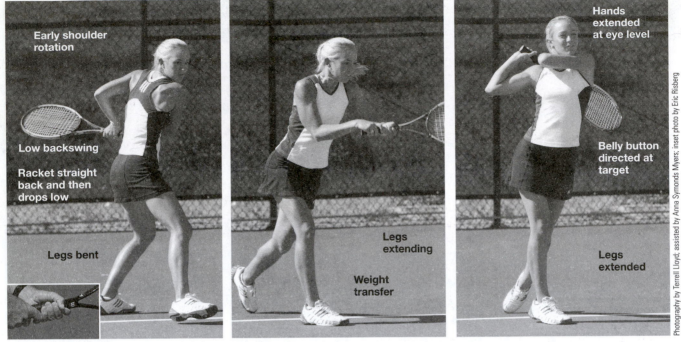

Early shoulder rotation

Low backswing

Racket straight back and then drops low

Legs bent

Photo 2.17A Backswing (two-hand backhand grip).

Legs extending

Weight transfer

Photo 2.17B Contact.

Hands extended at eye level

Belly button directed at target

Legs extended

Photo 2.17C Follow-through.

Photography by Terrell Lloyd; assisted by Anna Symonds Myers; inset photo by Eric Risberg

and the wrists firm. As with all strokes, the weight is transferred forward to the lead foot as the player steps into the ball to make contact off that lead foot (Photo 2.17B). The *follow-through* is a simple continuation of the stroke, with the legs extended, and the hands extended and at eye level, your belly button turned to your target. The full swing comes from your shoulders and requires a solid, compact swing action. The hands work together throughout the swing (Photo 2.17C).

Points to Remember

Two-Hand Backhand Groundstroke

1. Keep your arms close to your body throughout the stroke, and keep your wrists firm.

2. Make sure that the two hands are snug to each other on the grip.

3. Use a low backswing to a high follow-through.

4. Incorporate a compact, full swing.

Common Errors and How to Correct Them
(Two-Hand Backhand Groundstroke)

The Error	What Causes the Error	To Correct the Error
Stroking the ball into the net.	Hitting too far in front of the lead leg or not following the low-to-high pattern.	Hit off the lead leg, and follow through to a high position.
Hitting the ball long or high against the fence.	Dropping the racket to a low position and bending the knees in an exaggerated low-to-high follow-through and leg extension.	Swing low to high, and use a low leg bend followed by an extension of the legs, but eliminate the exaggerated movement.
Hitting the ball off the end of the racket or not getting to the ball in time.	Poor reaction time and little anticipation of where the ball will be hit.	Concentrate on the ball when it is in on the far side of the net. Remember that the radius of the reach is shorter with a two-hand backhand than with a one-hand backhand.

Synopsis of the Groundstroke

Groundstrokes are the basis of all play in tennis. The developing player has to grow with the game and progress from a stationary position of hitting groundstrokes to a moving situation that will allow setting up to hit a ball. To balance the skill aspect of hitting groundstrokes, the player has to work on both sides of the body equally to develop both forehand and backhand. The beginning player has to be skilled at simple tasks ranging from dropping a ball and hitting a groundstroke to knowing where home base is and moving from home base to retrieve and stroke the ball.

Learning how to *drop and hit the ball* to begin a rally is necessary if a player is going to practice, warm up, or actually play the game. In a forehand groundstroke, the drop should be toward the sideline and toward the net so the player has to extend the arm to reach the ball and step, transferring weight to the lead leg to hit the ball. Dropping the ball anywhere else would confuse the player, eliminate the same form development for each stroke, and provide a difficult setup to begin a rally. One of the reasons for a forehand developing more quickly is that the player practices more on the forehand side. This is because it is more convenient to drop the ball on that side to begin a rally (Photos 2.18A and B).

The drop for the backhand should be attempted as often as the forehand drop to encourage development of the backhand stroke. The backhand differs from the forehand drop only in that the drop is completed under the racket on the backhand side and the racket is not yet in a complete backswing position. The ball is dropped in a palm-up position, and a lifting action allows the ball to bounce and come straight back up off the rebound to midthigh level to be hit. During the drop and swing, the body is turned to the side, facing the appropriate sideline

Self-Drop For Forehand

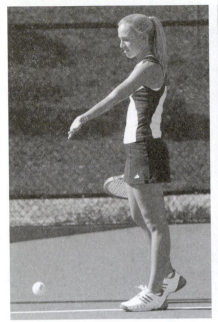

Photo 2.18A Drop the ball toward the sideline and toward the net.

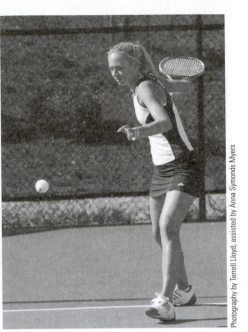

Photo 2.18B Ball should bounce and come straight back up to mid-thigh.

Self-Drop for Backhand

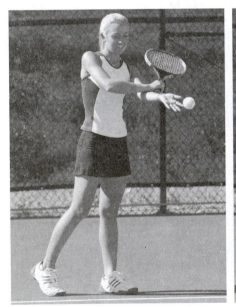

Photo 2.19A Drop the ball toward the sideline and toward the net.

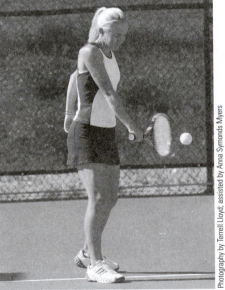

Photo 2.19B Ball should bounce and come straight back up to mid-thigh.

(Photos 2.19A and B). The drop for the two-hand backhand is the same as for the basic backhand except you need to re-grasp with your two-hand grip after dropping the ball.

Practice with groundstrokes usually begins from a stationary position. The area behind the baseline is known as **homebase** (Figure 2.1). It is a great learning experience for the player just beginning to develop the mechanics of a sound groundstroke to have all balls hit deep to that position. The rationale for having balls thrown to students in the early stages of skill development or having a ball machine toss balls directly to a player is to ensure that homebase is identified and that practice is as consistent as possible. There comes a time, however, when the player has to leave homebase and move after a ball hit a distance away. The player must leave the homebase area, move toward the ball, and hit a groundstroke—then return to homebase.

Moving to the ball, which involves proper footwork, is a major problem for the beginning tennis player. If the ball is hit deep with a high and deep bounce, the player must retreat behind the baseline to get to the ball, set up, then step back into the ball with good weight transfer. To respond to a deeply hit ball, the player first must turn the shoulder (remember—the player always starts from a ready position) and take a sideward step with the foot that is on the same side as the turning shoulder. From that point, the movement is either a sideward response or a total turn and run to at least a step behind and away from the ball. The turning movement must occur as soon as

Photography by Terrell Lloyd; assisted by Anna Symonds Myers

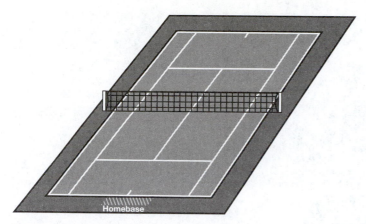

Figure 2.1 Homebase.

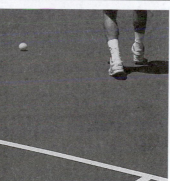

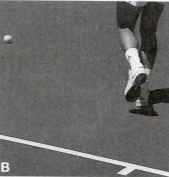

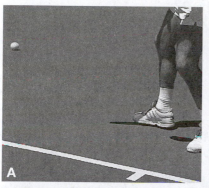

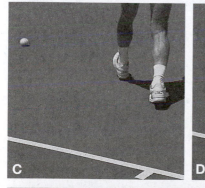

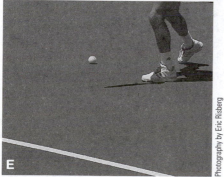

Photography by Eric Risberg

Photo 2.20 Footwork and moving to the ball hit beyond the baseline.

possible, preferably before the ball crosses the net (Photo 2.20).

Moving to the ball when it is in front of the player is a little easier, but it requires early anticipation of where the ball is going. The player moves in a direct line forward with timing that will provide opportunity to set up behind the ball and away from the line of the ball's flight. The last part of the movement involves slowing down and gathering the body in a controlled manner, then stepping in a direct line to the ball with the racket-side foot first, thereby aligning the body to the path of the ball and establishing the next sequential step.

The next step involves stepping into the ball with the non-racket-side leg in a timed movement to synchronize with the contact part of the full stroke. As the racket-side leg steps first, the racket is in a backswing position, then it comes through into the ball at contact (Photo 2.21). There is no difference between hitting a forehand and a backhand groundstroke. The point is to set up behind and to the side of the ball as described when hitting the ball to start a rally.

Moving to the ball or hitting from the baseline will be enjoyable if a foundation is built from the baseline that is consistent for all groundstrokes. The foundation of hitting with a stepping movement, having good weight transfer, and developing a sound stroke pattern is basic. The foundation must be repeated so often that each stroke becomes an instinctive reaction that does not require thought.

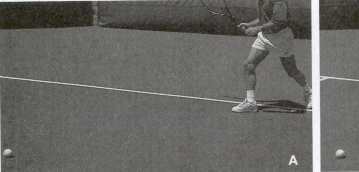

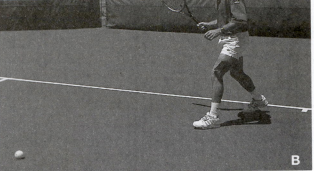

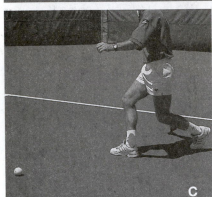

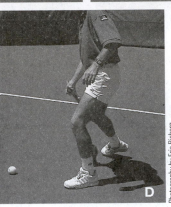

Photography by Eric Risberg

Photo 2.21 Footwork and moving to the ball hit in front of the baseline.

Increasing Beginner Skills: Forehand Groundstroke—Slice and Topspin

The basic forehand groundstroke is the stroke that beginners start with, but if they are to increase their skills, they have to identify and eventually hit a *forehand slice groundstroke* and a *forehand topspin groundstroke*. All three strokes are similar, but the **slice** requires a high backswing and a slightly open-face contact point, followed by a high follow-through (Photos 2.22A–C). The spin imparted to the ball is underspin, with the ball staying low to the net, followed by a skidding action, or low bounce, when rebounding off the court.

The **topspin** stroke begins with a very low backswing, a slightly closed racket face at contact, and a high follow-through. At contact the forearm rotates somewhat. In addition, the legs play a part in this stroke with a low bend of the knees during the backswing, followed by an extension of the legs in the follow-through position (Photos 2.23A–C). The spin of the ball is an overspin, or topspin, and the ball action upon striking the court surface is a high bounce. The grip used for a slice is still the eastern forehand grip, but to gain additional spin, the grip for the topspin changes to a more western grip.

The beginner has to first develop the basic stroke, then move to the slice and topspin in a progression. For most beginners, the slice is more difficult to develop. In contrast, the forehand topspin groundstroke comes naturally to many players, and now is typically the first forehand groundstroke that young players learn.

Forehand Slice Groundstroke

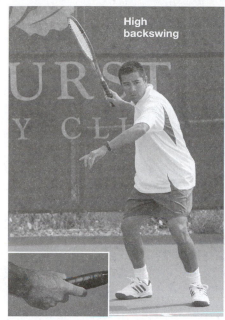
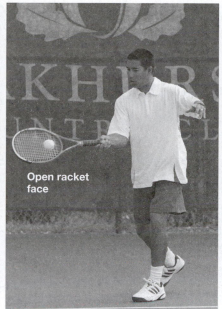

Photo 2.22A Backswing (eastern forehand grip).

Photo 2.22B Contact.

Photo 2.22C Follow-through.

Photography by Terrell Lloyd; assisted by Anna Symonds Myers; inset photo by Eric Risberg

Forehand Topspin Groundstroke

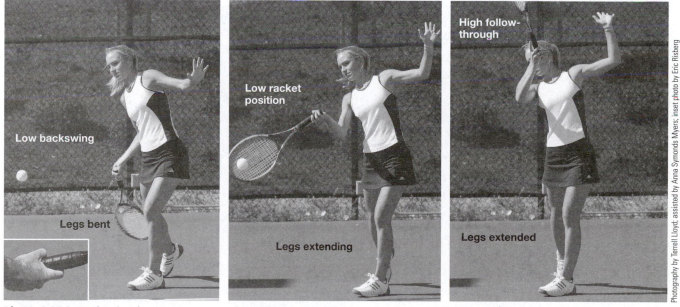

Photo 2.23A Backswing (western forehand grip).

Photo 2.23B Contact.

Photo 2.23C Follow-through.

Photography by Terrell Lloyd; assisted by Anna Symonds Myers; inset photo by Eric Risberg

Backhand Slice Groundstroke

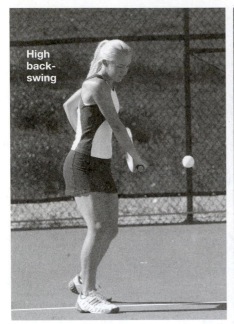
High back-swing

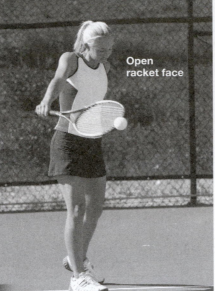
Open racket face

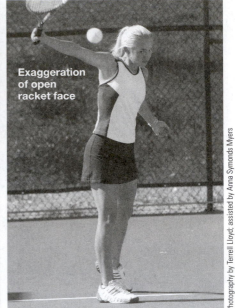
Exaggeration of open racket face

Photography by Terrell Lloyd; assisted by Anna Symonds Myers

Photo 2.24A Backswing.   **Photo 2.24B** Contact.   **Photo 2.24C** Follow-through.

Increasing Beginner Skills: Backhand Groundstroke—Slice and Topspin

As with the forehand slice and topspin groundstroke, the basic backhand is the starting point for a beginner. But two strokes add to the groundstroke development: the *backhand slice groundstroke* and the *backhand topspin groundstroke*. The slice is executed with a slightly high backswing, an open racket face at contact, and a high follow-through (Photos 2.24A–C). The ball action is the same underspin with a skidding action as it rebounds from the court. The eastern grip is used with this stroke.

The topspin groundstroke starts with a low backswing, a slightly closed face at contact, and a high follow-through (Photos 2.25A–C). The forearm does rotate slightly from contact to follow-through, and the legs bend and extend from backswing to follow-through. The eastern backhand grip is used for both the slice and the topspin.

A two-hand slice groundstroke has the same action as an eastern backhand slice stroke. And a two-hand backhand topspin stroke is particularly successful because the stroke is compact and already pro-grammed to begin low in the back-swing and continue on through to an extensive high follow-through. A two-hand backhand becomes particularly successful when hitting a topspin backhand because the stroke is compact and already pro-grammed to begin low in the back-swing and continue on through to an extensive follow-through.

Just as with the comments re-garding the forehand groundstroke, beginners have to start with the basic backhand and progress to spin strokes. Often the slice becomes an extremely reliable stroke for the de-veloping player, and the topspin can become quite lethal, particularly for a player who develops a two-hand backhand.

Backhand Topspin Groundstroke

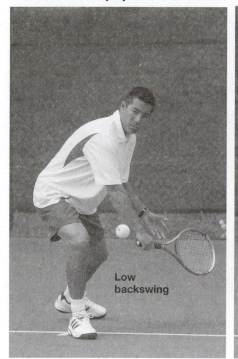

Low backswing

Photo 2.25A Backswing.

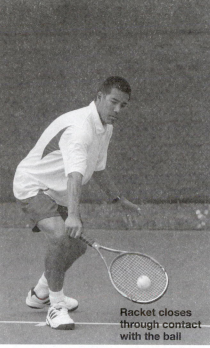

Racket closes through contact with the ball

Photo 2.25B Contact.

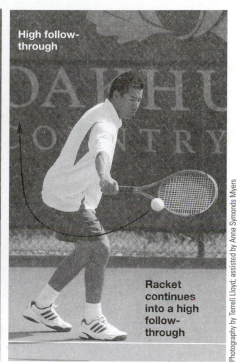

High follow-through

Racket continues into a high follow-through

Photo 2.25C Follow-through.

Photography by Terrell Lloyd; assisted by Anna Symonds Myers

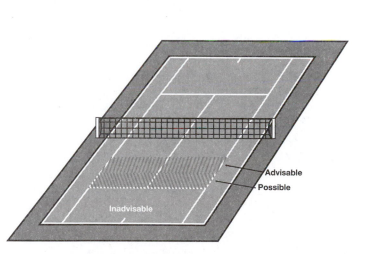

Advisable

Possible

Inadvisable

Figure 2.2 Foundation—when to go to the net, when to stay at homebase.

Increasing Beginner Skills: Using the Groundstroke to Hit an Approach Shot

Moving to hit a ball situated between the baseline and the net is related to foot movement and also to decision-making. It now is important to recognize which shots require the player to step into the ball, stroke the ball, then return to homebase, or to move up to the ball and hit it, then advance to the net. Shots that are hit at the service court line require the decision to continue to advance to the net to play a potential volley, or to retreat to homebase. Balls that are hit between the service court line and the net require no decision: The player is advised to move forward to play at the net (Figure 2.2). When a decision must be made to either attack the net or retreat to the baseline, or when the player must go to the net, a modification of the groundstroke called an *approach shot* is called for.

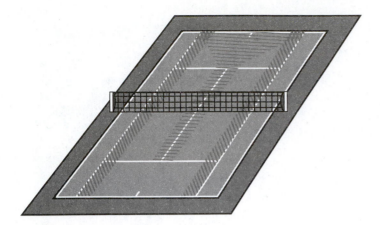

Figure 2.3 Approach shots down the line and in the corners.

When it is determined that a player is going to hit an approach shot, that player must develop certain perceptions. First, a player must realize that the approach shot is simply a groundstroke they must move toward in order to hit the ball. Second, the approach must be viewed as a gift given as a reward for excellent play on the baseline that forced the opponent to hit the ball short rather than deep. Third, a player must recognize that approach shots often allow for too much time to decide what to do with the ball, resulting in a shabby attempt at hitting an approach shot. Fourth, the approach shot must be considered a modified version of the full groundstroke swing. Fifth, as the beginning player improves, there is a transition from a basic stroke to a slice groundstroke.

The third and fourth concepts have to be discussed in more detail. Having time to hit a shot allows the player to decide how and where to hit the ball. There is a problem, however, when the player changes the decision once it has been made. The player must make one decision on *how* to hit the ball, and another on *where* to hit the ball (deep or at an angle). Both judgments are difficult for beginning players, and as a result, they simply bang away at the ball, usually missing everything but

the back fence. A player must be aware of the choices and continue to learn from mistakes, gaining confidence from each opportunity to hit an approach shot. The target areas are based on zones. An approach shot positioned on the side zones should be hit down that sideline; a shot positioned in the center zone should be hit down the center of the court or deep to either corner (Figure 2.3).

Modifying the approach shot to cope with the target area is the skill adaptation to the groundstroke. Three adaptations to the approach shot from the groundstroke are:

1. Shorten the backswing.

2. Visualize the target.

3. Select the appropriate shot sequence.

An approach shot doesn't require extensive force behind it, as does a shot from the baseline. Instead of bringing the racket back in a full backswing motion, it should be brought back perhaps two-thirds of that distance. If, when preparing to hit an approach shot, a player will develop mental imagery of the target as being located at the opponent's service court line, the ensuing distance the ball travels probably will increase by a third of the distance. As a result, the ball will really travel to the opponent's baseline. The baseline is the spot desired for a deep hit, but the mental imagery has to give a shortened target distance to allow for the shortened distance the ball actually must travel.

Selecting the appropriate shot is based on the position of the ball to be hit. Balls that are returned low are usually hit to the opponent's backhand, and the player then moves to the net to hit a volley off the opponent's assumed weaker backhand return. Returns that hit the center of the court have a target area of the corners. Hitting a ball cross-court that is positioned down the line opens up too much court for the opposing player to return successfully.

The player continues the sequence of moving from the baseline to hitting an approach shot by moving to the net to play a potential volley return of the opponent's reaction to the approach shot. Discussion of the volley sequence is found in Chapter 3.

Checkpoints ✔✔

1. The three parts to a basic forehand groundstroke are
   a. preparation, loop backswing, and follow-through.
   b. preparation, contact, and follow-through.
   c. loop backswing, contact, and follow-through.
   d. preparation, loop backswing, and contact.

2. When hitting a forehand groundstroke, the
   a. wrist and forearm remain firm but relaxed.
   b. wrist is laid back and the elbow is hyperextended.
   c. wrist remains firm with the elbow hyperextended.
   d. wrist is laid back and the elbow is firm but relaxed.

3. Correcting the error of shots hit short with little velocity requires
   a. changing the swing from slightly low to high.
   b. changing the swing from slightly high to low.
   c. transferring weight into the ball at contact.
   d. stepping away from the ball at contact.

4. To hit a topspin forehand groundstroke requires an adjustment from the basic stroke, which includes
   a. eastern grip, low-to-high swing, and leg flexion and extension.
   b. western grip, low-to-high swing, and leg flexion and extension.
   c. western grip, flat backswing to high follow-through, and leg flexion and extension.
   d. eastern grip, low-to-high swing, and leg flexion.

5. A characteristic of hitting a basic backhand groundstroke is
   a. shoulder leading into contact with racket rotating around the wrist and elbow leading the racket.
   b. shoulder leading into contact with the wrist and elbow leading the racket.
   c. shoulder held back with the wrist and elbow leading the racket.
   d. shoulder leading into contact with the racket rotating around the wrist and elbow.

6. A backhand groundstroke hit long is caused by
   a. hitting with poor timing and/or weight on the back foot.
   b. too much of an open racket face with no follow-through.
   c. hitting with an open racket face, poor timing, and not following through.
   d. all three of the above causes.

7. The two-hand backhand groundstroke requires that the follow-through is a
   a. racket finish in a wrap-around of shoulders and head, and the belly button turned toward the hitting target.
   b. racket finish high with the belly button turned toward the hitting target.
   c. racket finish in a wrap-around of shoulders and head, and the belly button turned to the racket side of the body.
   d. combination of *a*, *b*, and *c*.

8. Hitting the ball off the end of the racket when hitting a two-hand backhand is caused by
   a. not dropping the racket to a low position.
   b. poor reaction timing and limited anticipation.
   c. hitting too far out in front of the lead leg.
   d. not swinging low to high.

(continued)

Checkpoints ✔✔

(continued)

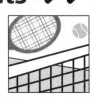

9. When attempting to hit a moving ball that is short or deep, the player must
   a. set up even with the ball and step up even with the ball to hit it.
   b. set up in front of the ball and step into the ball to hit it.
   c. move at an angle to set up behind the ball and step into the ball to hit it.
   d. move straight to the ball and step into the ball to hit it.

10. Approach shots should be hit
    a. with a visual image target to the opponent's service court line.
    b. with a reduced backswing.
    c. with a target of down-the-line to the corners and to the center.
    d. using *b* in combination with *a* and *c*.

Answers to Checkpoints can be found on page 147.

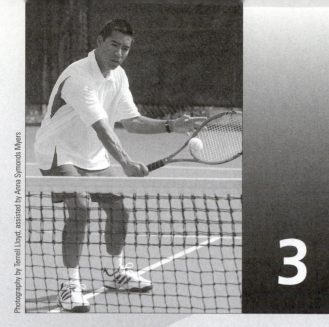

Photography by Terrell Lloyd; assisted by Anna Symonds Myers

3

Net Play

The volley is one of two strokes hit when the ball is in mid-air prior to striking the court on the bounce. It is an uncomplicated punching action stroke also described as a "blocking-the-ball action." The volley is used in singles play following an approach shot or in a serve-and-volley combination. In doubles, the volley also is used following an approach shot and as a serve-and-volley combination, and it is used with a player positioned at the net during a serve.

Early in their development all players must learn the skills involved in the volley. A singles player may avoid most situations involving the volley, but in doubles play there is no choice but to be located at the net on most shots played.

The volley shot begins from the *ready position* as described when preparing to hit a groundstroke, except that the racket is held higher, at chin level (Photo 3.1). From this position the player who is at the net may respond to either a forehand or a backhand volley. Part of the preparation in the ready position is to assume a grip that is both comfortable and functional.

The *continental grip* usually is recommended for the volley, as no adjustment has to be made for a forehand or a backhand volley (Photo 3.1). Often there is not enough time to change grips when at the net because of the high velocity of a ball and the short distance from the opposing player. The strength of the continental grip is that the backhand is firm and solid when punching the volley. The weakness is that the grip for a forehand provides a weaker base, forcing the player to adjust at the net by changing to an eastern forehand when time permits. Most successful players do "cheat" and move the hand on the grip for most volley shots, provided that they have the time to change and also to change back following the stroke.

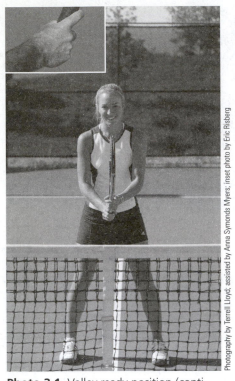

Photo 3.1 Volley ready position (continental grip).

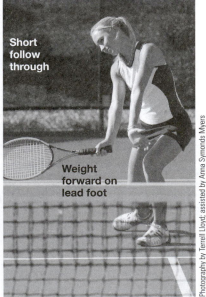

Forehand Volley

The *forehand volley* begins with a "short" backswing created by a shoulder turn. The racket head is located above the hand as the racket is taken back even with the racket shoulder (Photo 3.2A). The *preparation* is completed with the weight centered on the racket-side foot. The racket comes forward at *contact* with the ball, with the face of the racket striking the back of the ball squarely at the front of the lead leg (Photo 3.2B). A slight downward path of the stroke with a slightly open racket face imparts some underspin to the ball.

At contact the racket head is positioned above the hand, the wrist remains firm, and the grip also is firm to prevent the racket from turning in the hand at impact. A step is taken with the opposing leg, and the weight is transferred to that leg. The knees are bent from backswing to contact. It should be repeated that the racket must be in front of the lead leg at contact.

The *follow-through* (Photo 3.2C) is the final part of the punching action. A short downward motion, with the bottom edge of the racket leading, completes the stroke. The lead leg is still bent during follow-through, with the weight centered over that leg. Upon completing the follow-through, the player must return to a ready position in preparation for the next volley.

Forehand Volley Sequence

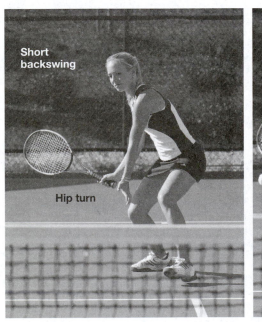

Short backswing

Hip turn

Photo 3.2A Preparation.

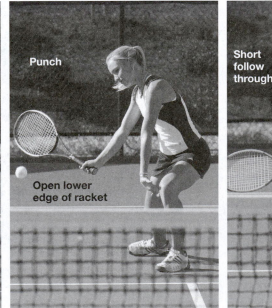

Punch

Open lower edge of racket

Photo 3.2B Contact with the ball.

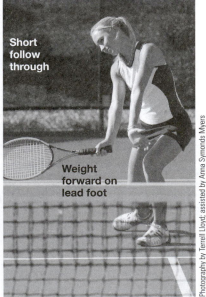

Short follow through

Weight forward on lead foot

Photo 3.2C Follow-through.

Photography by Terrell Lloyd; assisted by Anna Symonds Myers; inset photo by Eric Risberg

Photography by Terrell Lloyd; assisted by Anna Symonds Myers

Backhand Volley Sequence

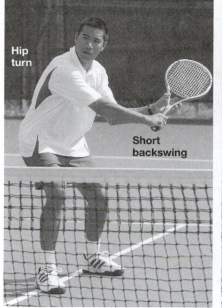

Hip turn

Short backswing

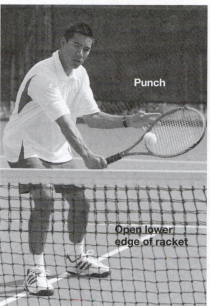

Punch

Open lower edge of racket

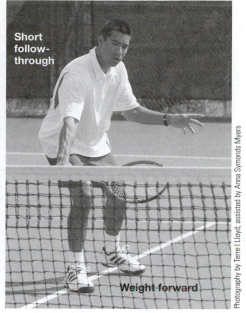

Short follow-through

Weight forward

Photography by Terrell Lloyd; assisted by Anna Symonds Myers

Photo 3.3A Preparation.   **Photo 3.3B** Contact with the ball.   **Photo 3.3C** Follow-through.

Backhand Volley

The *backhand volley* is executed like the forehand volley, but it is easier to complete mechanically because the shoulder turn is already to the backhand side and the elbow and shoulder work as a firm backboard when striking the ball. In *preparation*, the racket head is brought back to the non-racket side and is positioned above the hand. The weight of the body is centered over the non-racket-side foot, and the backswing is short with a firm wrist (Photo 3.3A).

At *contact*, the weight shifts forward to the racket leg as that leg steps into the ball. The racket face strings make full square contact with the back of the ball with a punching action that includes a firm wrist and arm and a firm grip on the racket. Contact is made slightly in front of the lead leg, with the racket above the hand (Photo 3.3B). The knees are bent from preparation through contact and into the follow-through.

The *follow-through* is a continuation of the punch action, with the bottom edge of the racket leading to apply a slight spin to the ball (Photo 3.3C). At the end of the follow-through, the weight is centered on the leading leg and the racket is extended a short distance forward. The recovery must be quick as the player returns to the ready position at the net.

Two-hand Backhand Volley

A *two-hand backhand volley* also can be used at the net. The stroke is the same as the basic *backhand volley*, but you are limited in terms of arm and leg extension. This is a relatively severe limitation, but with good footwork and the reminder to keep your arms into your body, it is an effective volley stroke (Photos 3.4A–C). As you develop confidence and skill at the net, you need to move away from two hands to a more effective one-hand backhand volley stroke.

Two-hand Backhand Volley Sequence

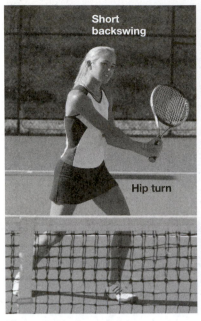

Photo 3.4A Preparation.

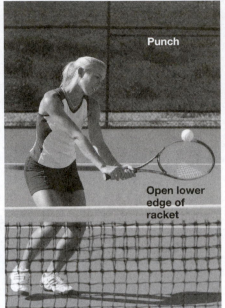

Photo 3.4B Contact with the ball.

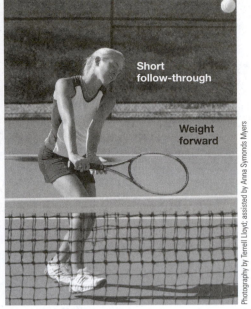

Photo 3.4C Follow-through.

Photography by Terrell Lloyd; assisted by Anna Symonds Myers

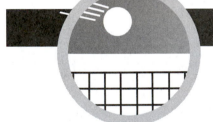

Points to Remember

Volley

1. Punch the ball—don't swing at it.
2. Keep the backswing and follow-through brief.
3. Keep the racket above the hand throughout the stroke.
4. Step into the ball if time allows.
5. Stay low on the ball.
6. Hit behind the ball, then follow through with the bottom edge of the racket leading.
7. Make contact in front of the lead leg.
8. Maintain control of the racket with a firm grip and firm wrist throughout the stroke.

Common Errors and How to Correct Them (Volley)

The Error	What Causes the Error	To Correct the Error
Balls that have no pace or just drop off the racket strings.	Not hitting in front of the lead leg; not transferring weight into the ball at contact.	Hit slightly in front of the lead leg between the body and the net. Step into and punch through the ball.
Racket turns in the hand, causing lack of control of the ball.	Lack of a firm grip, or grip size is too small.	Tighten the grip or increase the size of the grip for better control.
Ball strikes the net following contact.	Player not getting "down on the ball" and bending the knees when the ball is below the height of the net. Or racket face is not open enough at contact.	Bend the knees all the way through the shot. If the ball is below the net, open the racket face and punch through the ball.
Ball is hit long.	Elbow usually not firm.	Keep elbow away from the body through contact.

Increasing Beginner Skills: Insight When Hitting a Volley

Anticipation is a key to playing well at the net. If the player at the net is afraid of the ball, he or she cannot anticipate. If the player "sees" the ball early, reacting as the ball comes off the opposing player's racket rather than waiting until the ball arrives at the net, the volleying player will be effective at the net. Once the reaction has been improved, the next important phase is to attack by stepping into the ball rather than waiting for the ball to arrive at the net. Even guessing, as part of anticipation, is better than standing at the net and waiting.

Footwork for the volley is important to the stroke so form can be added to the total maneuver. Footwork enables the player to step into the ball with body weight behind the punch, and to move efficiently to get to the ball. The first part of the footwork involves a shoulder turn and hip pivot. From a ready position, the player should pivot the hips toward the anticipated position of the ball. With the hip turn, the shoulders will

turn also, and the racket-side foot will react by pivoting until the body weight centers over that foot.

Three basic ball positions presented to the volleyer are:

1. The setup with the shoulder and hip turn, involving a small cross-step.
2. The wide ball that forces the player to take a lengthened cross-step.
3. The ball hit at the player, which requires a defensive reaction.

The *setup* is initiated with the shoulder and hip turn, followed by the turn of the inside of the foot and a step forward and a little across the body with the opposite leg (Photos 3.5 and 3.6). The *wide ball* is reached by the same movement used for the setup, but the step across the body with the opposite leg requires an elongated, direct movement (Photos 3.7 and 3.8).

The *ball hit at the player* requires that the player hit with a backhand volley, if at all possible. The player

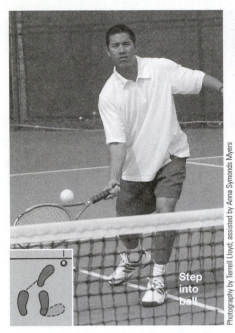

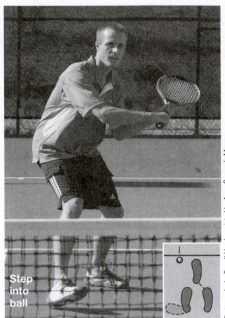

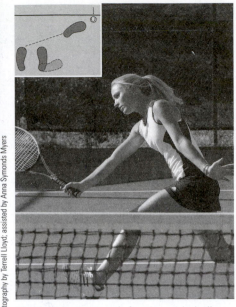

Photo 3.5 Footwork for the setup volley (forehand).

Photo 3.6 Footwork for the setup volley (backhand).

Photo 3.7 Footwork for the wide-ball volley (forehand).

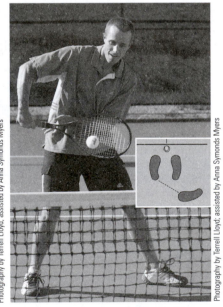

Photo 3.8 Footwork for the wide-ball volley (backhand).

Photo 3.9 Footwork for the ball hit at the net player (backhand).

must pivot off the racket foot and if there is time step with the non-racket foot behind the opposite foot to turn the shoulder sideways to the ball (Photo 3.9 diagram insert). The player then must lean back into the path of the ball (Photo 3.9).

Body elevation also is important to successfully complete the volley, as balls are not going to be returned at shoulder level in all situations. The legs must be either bent or extended for many of the volley stroke situations.

A *low volley* forces the player to bend the knees and get low to the ball (Photos 3.10 and 3.11). The hip and shoulder turn must occur to position the shoulder to the ball, and the legs must bend as low as possible. The volleyer steps into the ball with the opposite foot and punches under and through the ball, using underspin to lift the ball over the net. The underspin is achieved by opening the racket face. The closer the ball is to the court at contact, the more open the racket face should be. The follow-through of the low shot continues with an upward, short movement of the racket, with the knees remaining bent. Throughout the stroke, the racket should stay above the hand, if possible, to ensure proper technique and stroking action.

The *high volley* forces the volleyer to extend the body and the legs to reach the ball. The shoulder turn must occur early to permit the racket to be taken back a little farther and higher than for the basic volley.

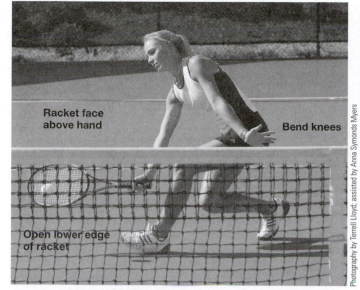

Racket face
above hand

Bend knees

Open lower edge
of racket

Photography by Terrell Lloyd; assisted by Anna Symonds Myers

Photo 3.10 Low forehand volley.

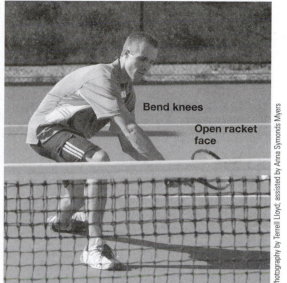

Bend knees

Open racket
face

Photography by Terrell Lloyd; assisted by Anna Symonds Myers

Photo 3.11 Low backhand volley.

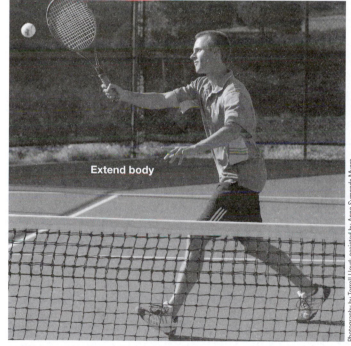

Extend body

Photography by Terrell Lloyd; assisted by Anna Symonds Myers

Photo 3.12 High forehand volley.

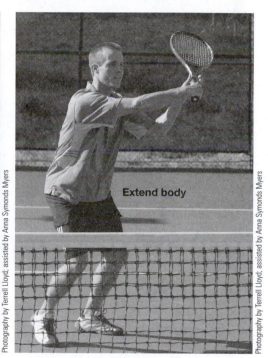

Extend body

Photography by Terrell Lloyd; assisted by Anna Symonds Myers

Photo 3.13 High backhand volley.

The player then steps into the ball with the opposite leg and punches down and through the ball. The follow-through moves in the direction of the ball just hit and ends at waist level. The punching pattern is a high-to-low closing stroke. The wrist is locked, and the stroke is firm (see Photos 3.12 and 3.13).

The volley has to be *incorporated into the total game* of the beginning player. At this point, the volley is an extension of the player hitting a groundstroke and advancing to the net, or hitting an approach shot and moving to the net, or hitting at the net in doubles play. The volley is a reward for forcing the opponent into a mistake, and it is executed best between the service court line and the net.

Beginning players will play most volleys off the net at a range of one to one and one-half racket lengths away from the net. More advanced players have a wider range back to the service court line, but the same players have the goal of moving closer to the net to be less vulnerable to a well-placed low shot at the feet.

Increasing Beginner Skills: Half Volley

Half volleys are necessary when the player is positioned in the midcourt area and is confronted with a return shot placed just in front of the feet. The player uses an eastern forehand or backhand grip, or a continental grip, and strokes the ball as a combination groundstroke and volley. The player must bend both legs to the extreme, with the lead leg bent at a right angle and the back leg nearly scraping the court surface.

The ball must be contacted on the "short" bounce or before it rises. The wrist is firm at contact, and the angle of the racket face is open just enough to permit the ball to clear the net. The backswing is short, as with an approach shot, and the follow-through lifts the body up from the low position. Throughout the shot, the head should stay down to ensure that the body does not lift early. The forehand half-volley contact point is at the lead leg, and the backhand point is in front of the lead leg (see Photos 3.14 and 3.15).

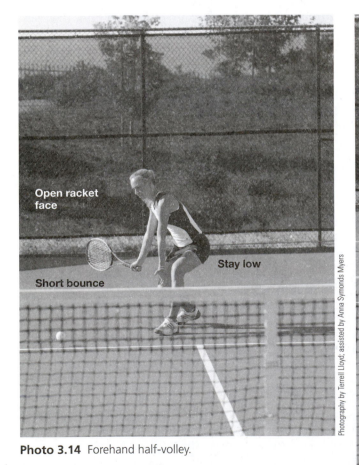

Open racket face

Short bounce

Stay low

Photography by Terrell Lloyd; assisted by Anna Symonds Myers

Photo 3.14 Forehand half-volley.

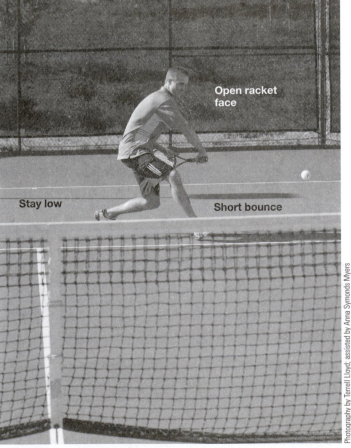

Open racket face

Stay low

Short bounce

Photography by Terrell Lloyd; assisted by Anna Symonds Myers

Photo 3.15 Backhand half-volley.

Checkpoints ✔✔

1. The type of grip used for the volley is the
   a. eastern forehand.
   b. eastern backhand.
   c. western forehand.
   d. continental.

2. The backswing for a volley shot is
   a. shortened.
   b. lengthened.
   c. the same as a regular ground-stroke.
   d. any of the three, depending on the situation.

3. Contact with the ball is made
   a. in front of the lead leg.
   b. behind the lead leg.
   c. even with the lead leg.
   d. with all three depending on the situation.

4. To correct the shot that hits the net following contact,
   a. tighten the grip.
   b. align the wrist, arms, and shoulders in a firm position.
   c. bend the knees through the shot.
   d. close the racket face.

5. The body position for a ball hit directly at the body of the volley-ing player is to
   a. use a backhand volley.
   b. drop step to hit the ball.
   c. use a forehand stroke.
   d. use *a* and *b* in combination with each other.

6. A low volley position requires
   a. opening the racket face at contact.
   b. closing the racket face at contact.
   c. hitting with a square face at contact.
   d. hitting off the back foot.

7. The beginning player has a comfort zone range at the net
   a. of 1 to 1 ½ racket lengths from the net.
   b. from the service court to the net.
   c. of 2 to 2 ½ racket lengths from the net.
   d. of anywhere on the court.

8. A half volley is hit with
   a. an open racket face at the top of the ball bounce.
   b. a closed racket face off a short bounce.
   c. a square face off a short bounce.
   d. an open face off a short bounce.

Answers to Checkpoints can be found on page 147.

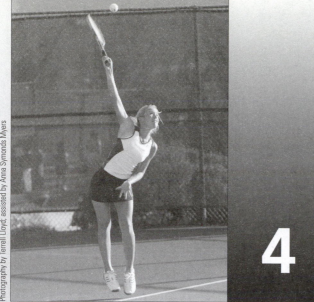

4

Service and Service Return

The service and service return are critical to success in tennis. Groundstroke skill enables the developing player to rally from the **baseline**. Without the skills of service and service return, the beginning player is not able to place the ball into play or to return a service for an actual game, set, or match. The three services that are used widely in tennis are: (1) the basic flat service, (2) the slice service, and (3) the topspin service. Discussion in this chapter will be limited to the flat serve as the basic beginner serve, and the slice serve as a serve to increase the beginner's skill.

Basic Flat Service

The *basic flat service* is a model for the service. A *service stance* is used in all serves. The feet are approximately shoulder-width apart, with the lead foot positioned approximately the length of a tennis ball from the baseline and the center mark of the baseline. The shoulder is pointed toward the service court target, the knees are slightly flexed, and the body from the waist up is upright (Photo 4.1).

The *grip* for the *flat service* (and for the two other services) is the

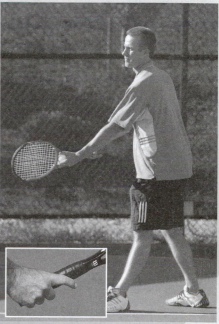

Photo 4.1 Service stance (continental grip).

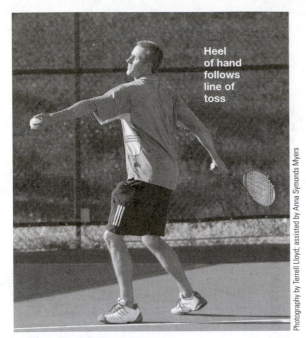

Heel
of hand
follows
line of
toss

Photography by Terrell Lloyd; assisted by Anna Symonds Myers

Photo 4.2 Beginning of toss.

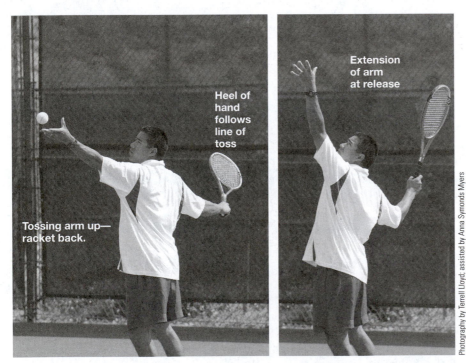

Heel of
hand
follows
line of
toss

Tossing arm up—
racket back.

Extension
of arm
at release

Photography by Terrell Lloyd; assisted by Anna Symonds Myers

Photo 4.3A Release.

Photo 4.3B Height of toss.

forehand grip, but you should change to a continental grip as soon as possible.

Skill is involved in *holding the ball for the toss* that initiates the serve action and also in *actually tossing the ball.* To begin any service, you must have two tennis balls in your possession. Keep one ball in the pocket of your tennis shorts so you have to deal with only one ball during any one serve.

Grasp the ball to be tossed with the fingertips and the thumb, with the heel of the hand pointing in the direction of the toss (Photo 4.2). From the support base, the ball is placed into a position off the lead shoulder between the player and the sideline, and higher than the reach of the racket. A straight arm lifts the ball from the waist to above the head. The heel of the hand is raised during the full arm movement. As the tossing arm begins the upward movement, the racket arm brings the racket back in synchronization with the toss. At the extension of the arm reach, the ball is released, culminating the lifting action. The toss must be executed the same way again and again so you can become consistent (Photos 4.3A and B).

When first learning the service, keep the feet shoulder-width apart throughout the serve. Initially, stability is more important than extra rhythm. Although the feet will not come together in the early stages of learning, the back foot will come forward automatically as the weight transfers toward the target on the follow-through (Photos 4.4A–C).

The first timing aspect of the service is the *toss synchronization as preparation for the service.* As the tossing hand begins the upward lift of the ball, the racket begins a backward movement with the arm straight. The two arms move in opposition. The racket continues back, with the elbow bending as the racket approaches the shoulder-blade area. The back of the elbow is at a right angle, and the arm is in an overhand throwing position. As the

continental, with some possible slight variations. The continental grip provides a flat surface for a square contact point. When learning to serve, you may begin by using an eastern forehand or a western

Footwork for Service

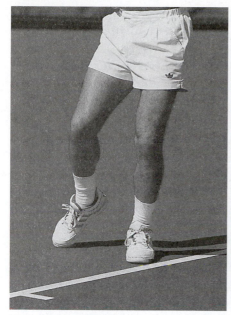

Photo 4.4A Backswing.

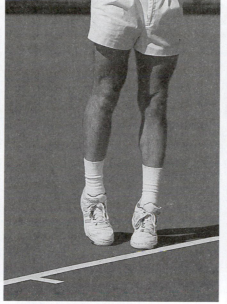

Photo 4.4B Contact.

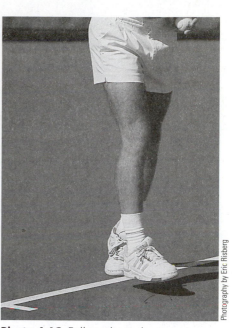

Photo 4.4C Follow-through.

Photography by Eric Risberg

ball reaches the top of the placement and begins to fall, the tossing hand will drop away and the hitting elbow will stay in a right-angle position (see Photos 4.5A–C).

Following the backswing, the initiation of contact occurs. The legs straighten from a bent position in preparation for bringing the racket through in a striking position, with the wrist and forearm breaking, and along with the shoulders, rotating through the contact of the ball. The arm and body are stretched fully. The back and top of the ball is hit with the racket face at about 4 inches down from the height of the toss. The body, led by the shoulder, opens up to the position of the ball at contact (Photo 4.5D).

The follow-through continues as momentum carries the racket through the ball and on down to the far non-racket-side leg. A definite weight transfer occurs during follow-through, with the momentum of the racket side pulling the body down and forward. This forces the back foot at the last moment to step forward for a balanced finish (Photo 4.5E).

The basic flat service is designed mechanically to hit through and down on the ball. The ball cannot be hit directly down in a straight line unless the server is at least 6'7" tall. The racket makes an upward movement at contact, followed by a breaking of the wrist and forearm through the ball. Most beginning players have a great desire to hit the flat serve as hard as they can, assuming that the idea is to hit the service with blazing speed. The problem is that few balls are placed accurately into the appropriate **service court**, which, in turn, means that the ball isn't placed in play to begin a point. This takes away from the fun of playing the game and minimizes the possibility for success. The idea is to hit a firm, controlled, rhythmical service that is placed in the service court effectively. Rhythm and ball placement are far more effective than a sometimes accurate, high-velocity serve.

Executing a full service versus a half-service requires discussion. Some beginning instruction starts with the racket already positioned between the server's shoulder blades

Flat Service

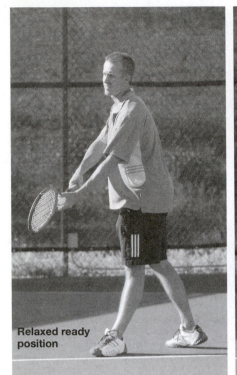

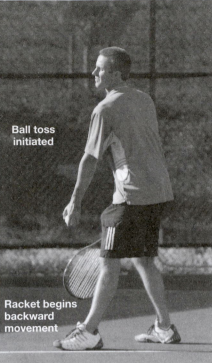

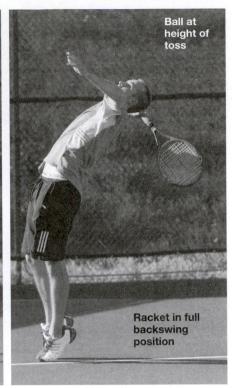

Photo 4.5A Ready position.

Photo 4.5B Initiation of release of ball and take back of racket.

Photo 4.5C Backswing continuation in preparation sequence.

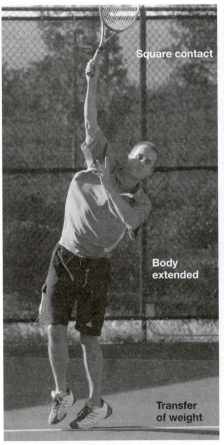

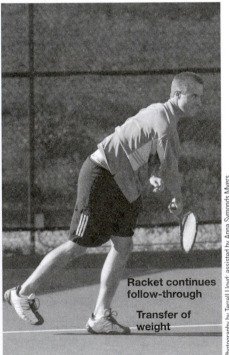

Photo 4.5D At contact.

Photo 4.5E Follow-through sequence.

Photography by Terrell Lloyd; assisted by Anna Symonds Myers

to eliminate the initial take-back portion of the stroke preparation. The purpose is to keep the stroke as simple as possible and not complicate coordination of the stroke.

The choice of a full serve versus a half-serve is a simple one of efficiency. Some highly skilled players use a half-service position, and many less skilled players use a full service. Some players are more comfortable initially with a full-service sequence, but all players need to see the half-service position to understand the upward position of the elbow and the location of the racket during the backswing to permit accurate timing of the stroke.

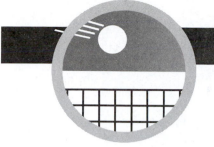

Points to Remember

Basic Flat Serve

1. Use the continental grip as soon as possible.
2. Time the toss with the take-back of the racket.
3. Keep your tossing arm straight, with the heel of the hand lifting in the direction of the toss, and releasing the ball at the extension of the arm.
4. Make the toss higher than the racket can reach.
5. Coil the body by arching your back and bending your knees during preparation.
6. Bring the racket through the ball with a slight upward wrist, followed by a downward wrist and forearm break, and shoulder turn.
7. Let your weight transfer carry your body and racket forward in the direction of the ball, with your back foot coming forward to regain balance.
8. Make sure the racket follows on through to the non-racket-side hip.

Common Errors and How to Correct Them (Basic Flat Serve)

The Error	What Causes the Error	To Correct the Error
Erratic placement of the serve.	Inconsistent toss.	Toss the ball by placing it off the lead shoulder between the shoulder and the sideline at a height above the reach of the racket.
Balls served short.	Ball hit too far out in front of the server toward the net; or server attempting to hit over ball; or ball too low at contact.	Toss the ball off the lead shoulder, at a height above the reach of the racket and between the server and the sideline. Focus on brushing through the back and top of the ball.
Ball toss goes behind the head.	Not lifting in a straight line with the tossing arm.	Use the heel of the hand as the lifting agent, along with a straight arm, thereby giving direction to the ball.
Ball served long.	Racket under the ball at contact, pushing the ball up; trying to hit the ball too hard.	Toss the ball off the lead shoulder, at a height above the reach of the racket and between the server and the sideline. Focus on brushing through the back, top of the ball at contact.
Stepping on the baseline during the serve.	Toss is too far over baseline toward net, or player steps with foot as if throwing a ball.	Toss the ball by laying it off the lead shoulder between the shoulder and the sideline at a height above the reach of the racket. Keep the lead foot firmly on the court.

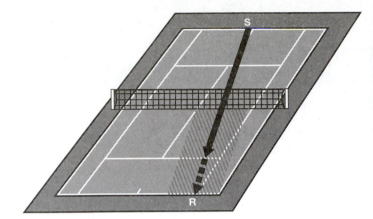

Figure 4.1 Return of serve position.

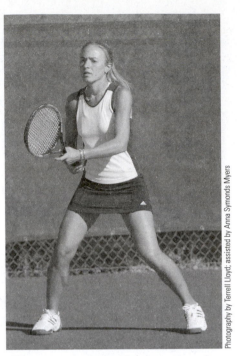

Photo 4.6 Ready position for return of serve.

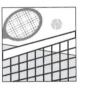

Return of Service

Because serves have different velocities, trajectories, and spins, the beginning player may be confronted with a series of decisions on how to cope with each type of serve.

Return of serve positioning is a matter of mathematics. The receiver must split the court in half in a line from the server to the receiver (Figure 4.1). The receiver cannot overplay to the side, attempting to return all serves with a forehand, because a server with a wide, flat serve or an adequate slice serve can place a ball that will kick off the court and out of reach of the player. It is much better for the receiver to position with the potential to hit either a forehand or a backhand equally.

The depth of the receiver's position depends on the velocity of the ball. If a player pushes the ball when serving and simply gets the ball in play, the receiver can move up and stand inside the baseline about halfway between the baseline and the service court line. If the server has a strong serve with high velocity, the receiver should stand at or slightly behind the baseline.

Returning the served ball effectively requires a special set of skills. First, the receiver should develop a relaxed attitude and appropriate ready position. The ready position (Photo 4.6), should be high to permit quick lateral movement and enable the receiver to hit through the ball with minimal adjustment. As the serve is hit, the receiver has to rotate the shoulders to a hitting position at the earliest possible moment. The receiver then must transfer weight into the stroke by stepping into the ball at contact.

The player also has to adopt a volley concept to the stroke. The backswing and follow-through have to be shortened to a movement longer than a volley but shorter than

Return of Serve: Forehand

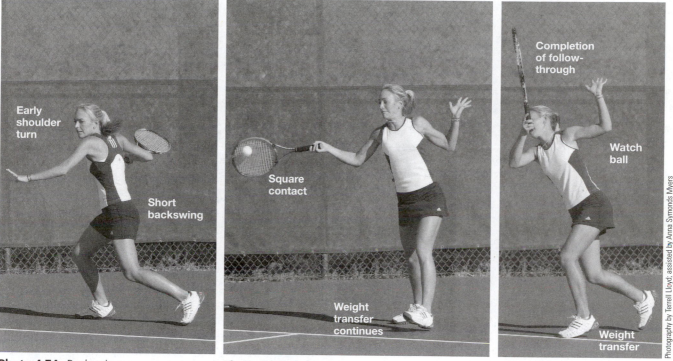

Photo 4.7A Backswing.

Photo 4.7B Contact.

Photo 4.7C Completion of follow-through.

a groundstroke. The shortened backswing enables the receiver to control the racket and bring it through in time to contact the ball. The action of the racket is more of a blocking or punching movement that pushes the ball back across the net, reversing the velocity of the serve.

The racket should be square to the ball and a little out in front of the lead leg, with a short follow-through to add direction to the ball. The racket should be held firmly throughout the stroke, particularly at contact. Finally, the receiver must watch the ball as long as possible up to the point of contact. Return of serve follows the same process and skill pattern whether hitting a forehand (Photos 4.7A–C) or backhand (Photos 4.8A–C). Selecting which side to hit from depends on the spin and direction of the ball and a responsive early rotation of the shoulders based on anticipating the position of the ball.

Target for return of serve is a moot point if the return player is just trying to get the racket on the ball. But with a degree of skill at returning a serve, the receiver can return the ball to spots on the court. The first consideration is where *not* to place the ball. Balls hit short to the server reward that server, so short returns should be eliminated. Serves that pull a return player off the court should be returned down the sideline rather than cross-court, and most returns hit soft and "up" should be avoided. If the receiver can remember to return deep with pace and velocity on the ball, subsequent play should enable the receiver to gain equal footing in a baseline rally.

Anticipation of the serve is both a physical and a mental exercise in the return of service. The receiver must look at the server's body language and concentrate on the ball. The body language will provide clues to the spin and velocity of the ball. If the server's racket-face pattern is to the outside of the ball and the toss is short and back toward

Return of Serve: Backhand

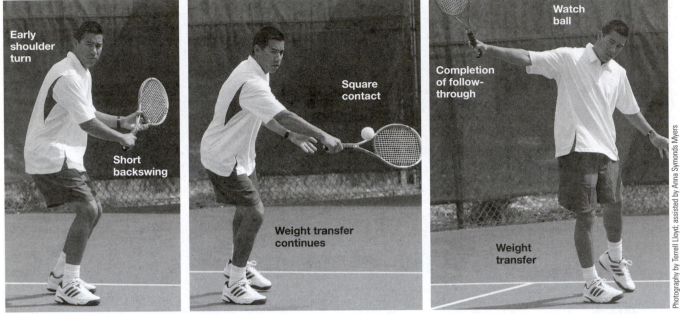

Photo 4.8A Backswing. **Photo 4.8B** Contact. **Photo 4.8C** Follow-through.

the racket shoulder, the serve will be a slice. If the toss is off the lead shoulder and toward the net, the ball will be a flat serve. A topspin serve will be interpreted by a toss above the head and/or more back arch than usual.

Velocity of the ball can be observed to some extent by the server's effort. Concentrating on the seams of the ball will permit the receiver to react physically to the direction of the ball. The mental efforts all combine to allow the receiver to make an early shoulder turn and pivot of the feet, thereby placing the racket in a backswing position.

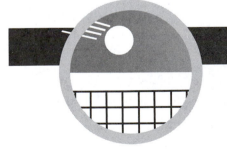

Points to Remember

Return of Serve

1. Throughout the serve, concentrate on the server's body language and on the ball.
2. Get the racket back early.
3. Be aggressive and step into the ball at contact.
4. Use a compact swing with a short backswing and follow-through.
5. Maintain a firm grip on the racket at contact.
6. Hit deep on all returns of serve.
7. Block all high-velocity serves.

Common Errors and How to Correct Them (Return of Serve)

The Error	What Causes the Error	To Correct the Error
Hitting the ball out beyond the server's baseline.	Swinging with a full groundstroke swing.	Use a compact swing; block high-velocity serves.
Pulling the ball across the court to the sidelines.	Racket contact with the ball too far out in front of the projected contact point.	Judge the velocity of the ball, and time your swing.
Ball coming off the racket late with direction toward the near sideline.	Not anticipating early and, as a result, not getting the shoulders turned and the racket back early.	Watch the ball, and react by turning the shoulders and pivoting the feet.
Cannot control direction of the ball.	Wrist isn't firm and grip isn't tight.	Keep a firm wrist and grip at contact.

Increasing Beginner Skills: Slice Service

A slice serve is often considered to be an intermediate skill, but in reality it can be taught as a beginning serve. Actually, it may be an easier serve for a beginner to learn.

The slice service puts a sidespin action on the ball, and it usually is used as a second serve in singles and a first and second serve in doubles. The spin permits the server to hit with greater accuracy and still place the serve deeply. A sidespin is imparted by contacting the back and side of the ball in sequence. The racket grip is a continental grip, and as more spin is needed, the grip can be adjusted to an eastern backhand grip. The result is that the ball lands in the court and kicks away from the the server's position.

The *slice service differs from the flat service* in the toss position and in the racket's movement pattern. The toss is the same distance from the body, but with less height (one of the advantages in the wind is a lower toss with a slice service). The ball is tossed between the lead shoulder and the middle of the body. More spin and less velocity is achieved

the closer the toss is to the back of the racket shoulder.

The difference between the slice and flat serve toss is that the flat serve toss is above the reach of the racket, as compared to the shorter toss for a slice service, and the toss is off the lead shoulder instead of between the lead shoulder and the middle of the body (Photos 4.9A–B and 4.10A–B for comparison).

During a slice service, contact is made on the side and back of the ball just below center, with the racket moving from high to low. The wrist and forearm move through a controlled motion and forceful action at contact. The shoulders are turned more with a slice service, leaving the body even more open at contact than with the flat service (Photos 4.11 and 4.12 for a comparison of flat serve versus slice serve).

The *full sequence of the slice service,* including the exceptions identified, is a rhythmical one with the take-away, followed by contact with the ball, and culminating with a follow-through down off the hip of the non-racket side. The weight

Toss for Flat Serve

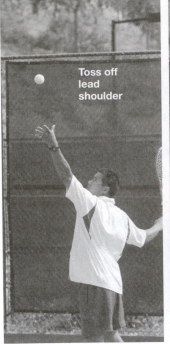

Toss off lead shoulder

Photo 4.9A Toss off lead shoulder.

Photo 4.9B Toss above the reach of racket.

Photography by Terrell Lloyd; assisted by Anna Symonds Myers

Toss for Slice Serve

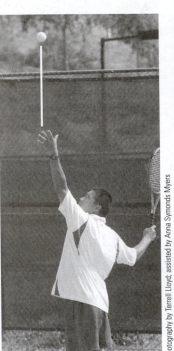

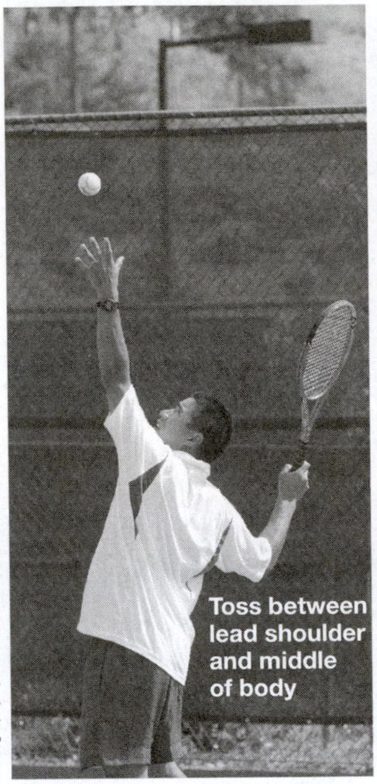

Toss between lead shoulder and middle of body

Photo 4.10A Toss between lead shoulder and middle of body.

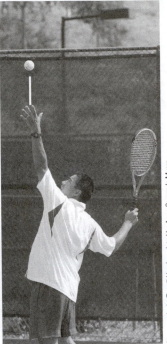

Photo 4.10B Short toss.

Photography by Terrell Lloyd; assisted by Anna Symonds Myers

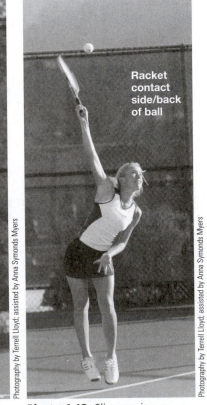

Racket contact at top back of ball

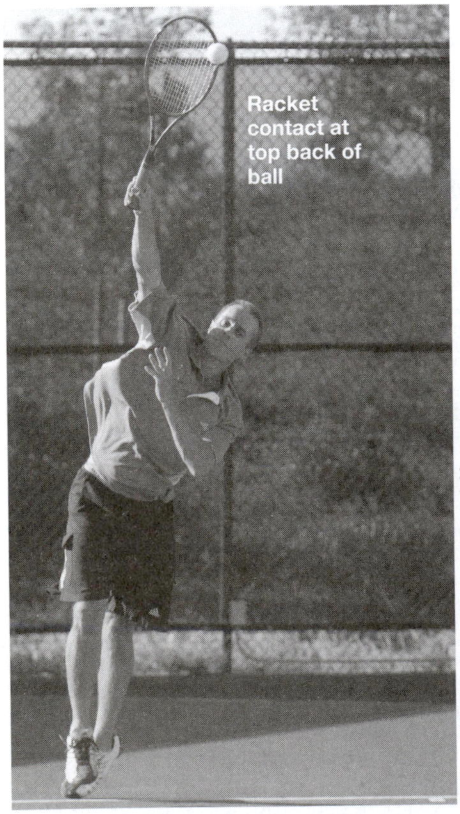

Photo 4.11 Flat service contact.

Photography by Terrell Lloyd; assisted by Anna Symonds Myers

Racket contact side/back of ball

Photo 4.12 Slice service contact.

Photography by Terrell Lloyd; assisted by Anna Symonds Myers

transfer is an aid to that sequence, as is the leg bend followed by extension of the leg at contact (Photos 4.13A–D).

A *summary of the differences and commonalities* of the two services may be helpful to the developing player. The differences, related to ball-toss position, racket-pattern movement, and foot position on the baseline, are outlined in Table 4.1. The commonalities involve weight transfer, elbow position on the backswing, and follow-through off the non-racket-side hip.

An additional commonality that will enhance the rhythm and timing of the total stroke is a change in foot movement from preparation through contact for the developing player. Instead of maintaining stability with a stationary foot position, the developing player may bring the back foot up even with the lead foot as the racket pattern begins to close on the ball at contact. This small change should be utilized when the player has developed balance and stroke timing from a more stationary position.

Slice Serve

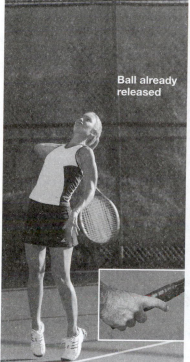

Photo 4.13A Backswing (continental grip).

Ball already released

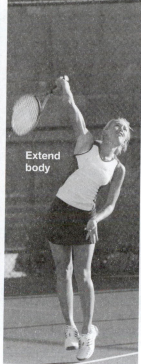

Extend body

Photo 4.13B Continuation of backswing.

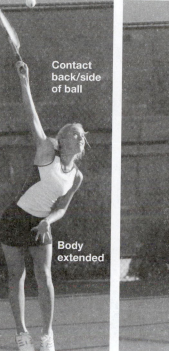

Contact back/side of ball

Body extended

Photo 4.13C Contact.

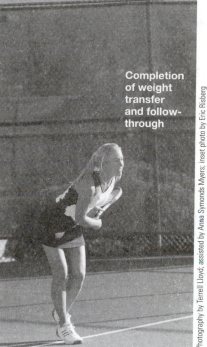

Completion of weight transfer and follow-through

Photo 4.13D Completion of follow-through.

Photography by Terrell Lloyd; assisted by Anna Symonds Myers; inset photo by Eric Risberg

Table 4.1 Differences Between the Two Major Services

Type of Service	Ball Toss Placement	Foot Position on Baseline	Racket Pattern Movement	Contact Position on Ball
Flat	off lead shoulder, above racket reach	even	straight through	back-top
Slice	between lead shoulder and racket shoulder, lower than racket reach	back foot slightly back	curving line	back-side just below center

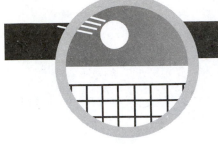

Points to Remember

Slice Serve

1. Use a continental grip.

2. Open the serving stance more than with the flat service.

3. Toss the ball lower than with the flat service, and toss more toward the back shoulder to obtain more spin.

4. Contact the ball sequentially on the back and side below center.

5. Transfer your weight forward through the sequence of the service, allowing the back foot to move forward to regain balance after contact.

Common Errors and How to Correct Them (Slice Serve)

The Error	What Causes the Error	To Correct the Error
Lack of spin on the ball.	Toss not far enough back to the racket shoulder; no continental grip; body doesn't open to the ball.	Toss between the two shoulders; check to make sure the grip is continental; or turn the lead shoulder more through the stroke.
Pulling the ball out of the serving court.	Turning the non-racket shoulder into the ball too early, and pulling the shoulder too far through the ball.	Point the non-racket shoulder to the service court target area from contact through follow-through, thereby reducing excessive shoulder turn.
A great amount of spin, but little velocity or distance.	Hitting the ball too far back on back shoulder, or racket pattern too far to the outside of the ball at contact.	Move toss toward the lead shoulder and/or control racket pattern through a sequential brushing action of the back and side of the ball.
Hitting the ball off the racket edge.	Too much of an eastern backhand grip.	Use a continental grip.

Checkpoints ✔✔

1. The toss for serve is a key to success. It should be executed
   a. by grasping the ball with the finger tips and thumb.
   b. with the heel of the hand pointed in the direction of the toss.
   c. by a straight lifting action of the arm.
   d. by using all three of the above skills.

2. The toss synchronization requires
   a. the racket beginning a backward movement as the tossing hand lifts.
   b. the racket placed in the middle of the shoulder blades as the tossing hand lifts.
   c. the racket beginning backward movement as the toss reaches its top height.
   d. use of all three of the above techniques.

3. The racket follow-through
   a. continues on a downward pattern finishing off the non-racket leg.
   b. continues on a downward pattern finishing off the racket leg.
   c. stops at waist level.
   d. can be any of the three depending on the type of serve used.

4. Weight of the body should
   a. be transferred forward by stepping with the lead foot.
   b. be centered at contact with the ball.
   c. rest on the back foot at contact with the ball.
   d. be transferred forward at contact with the ball.

5. The cause of the ball being consistently served into the net is
   a. that the toss is too high.
   b. that the server is attempting to hit over the ball.
   c. that the ball toss is too far out in front of the server.
   d. any of the three causes listed above.

6. The contact position on the ball for a slice serve is
   a. top-back.
   b. side-back.
   c. top.
   d. side.

7. The position of the ball on the toss for a slice serve is
   a. off the lead shoulder.
   b. off the racket shoulder.
   c. between the lead shoulder and the racket shoulder.
   d. any of the three positions.

8. A lack of spin applied to the ball when hitting a slice serve is caused by
   a. the toss being placed not far enough back toward the racket shoulder.
   b. turning the racket shoulder into the ball too soon.
   c. too extreme continental grip.
   d. contact on the side of the ball.

9. The return of serve ready positioning should be
   a. with the receiver standing to the forehand side of the line of the serve.
   b. with the receiver standing 2–4 feet inside the baseline.
   c. with the receiver standing 2–4 feet behind the baseline.
   d. with the receiver splitting the court in half in a line from the server to the receiver.

10. The correction for hitting a return of serve long is
    a. to use a compact swing and swing through the ball.
    b. to use a compact swing and block all serves.
    c. to use a compact swing and block all high-velocity serves.
    d. to use a full swing.

Answers to Checkpoints can be found on page 147.

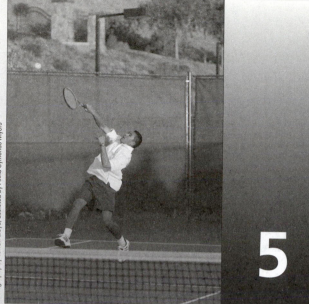

Photography by Terrell Lloyd; assisted by Anna Symonds Myers

5

Aerial Game

The lob and overhead combinations are basic strokes for the beginning player. Each skill complements the other in tennis. The lob is an extension of the groundstroke, discussed in Chapter 2, and the overhead is an elaboration of the service, discussed in Chapter 4. Overheads are attacking weapons. Lobs are used to react to an opponent playing at the net.

Overheads

The basic overhead is executed as a flat serve from the half-swing position. The overhead also can be executed from the forehand or the backhand side, but typically players run around the backhand to play a forehand overhead. The two forehand overheads in tennis are the simplistic orthodox overhead with little foot movement and a simple swing, and the more complex overhead (also termed "overhead with scissors kick") characterized by additional agility and timing (Photo 5.1). The orthodox overhead is the only overhead to be discussed here. The eastern forehand or continental grip is used for all forehand overheads.

The *orthodox forehand overhead* is a simple transition from the flat service. The player must maneuver underneath the ball that is hit as a lob, and from that position bring the racket back to the middle of the shoulder blades with the racket elbow at a right angle. The position of the racket physically touching between the shoulder blades provides a reference point for the player hitting the overhead. When the racket moves to a ready position, the simultaneous reaction is for the player to point to the ball with the non-racket arm and hand as a second reference point. The line of flight of the ball is similar to the ball toss, but the ball falls more rapidly and at a slightly different angle. The feet are shoulder-width apart, and the non-racket shoulder has turned to face the net and the intended target area (Photo 5.2).

In executing the overhead, the player's body is coiled and gathered, ready to time the stroke. The ball is hit off the lead shoulder, with the legs extending and the body uncoiling. Contact of racket to ball involves an up-and-over motion, providing a little topspin for greater net clearance and depth. The racket comes through the ball with a wrist break

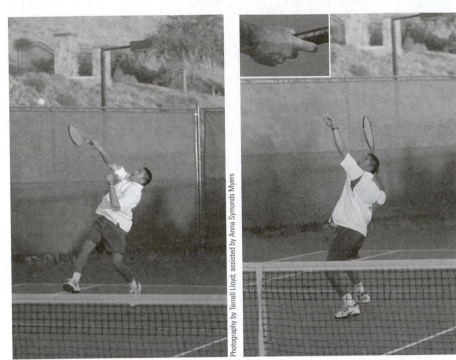

Photography by Terrell Lloyd; assisted by Anna Symonds Myers

Photo 5.1 Complex overhead.

Photography by Terrell Lloyd; assisted by Anna Symonds Myers; inset photo by Eric Risberg

Photo 5.2 Orthodox overhead (eastern forehand or continental grip).

and a follow-through to the far hip, but the action is shortened to accommodate the return of a ready position for the next shot (Photos 5.3A–D).

The full stroke is simplistic, eliminating wasted motion and extraneous actions. The feet remain stable until the follow-through pulls the back foot forward to catch the balance of the player at completion of the follow-through. The player is encouraged to hit out on the ball with smooth, rhythmical timing and control.

Advancing to more agility with the forehand overhead requires adding a few parts to the stroke. First, the player has to set up to hit the overhead. That movement consists of long, running strides to get to the general area as fast as possible and thereby allow time to set up the stroke. Once in the general area, the player will be situated behind the anticipated drop of the ball. At this point, the player takes small steps to adjust to the position of the ball. Balls that are hit over the player's head are handled in the same manner: taking long strides to get behind the ball, then short steps

Orthodox Forehand Overhead

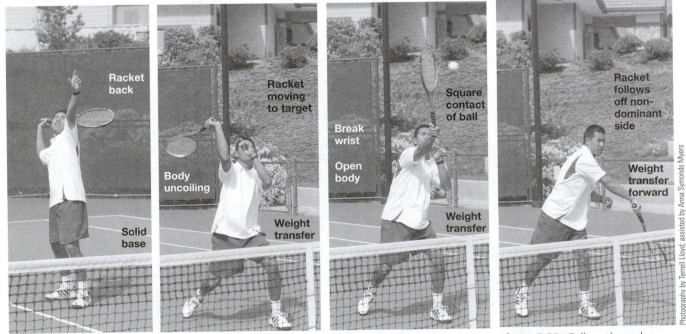

Photography by Terrell Lloyd; assisted by Anna Symonds Myers

Photo 5.3A Preparation. **Photo 5.3B** Initiation of swing. **Photo 5.3C** Contact. **Photo 5.3D** Follow-through.

Backhand Overhead

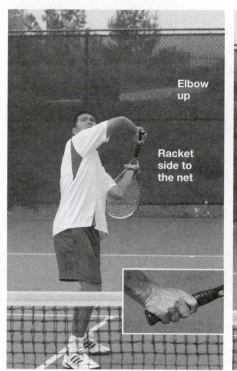

Photo 5.4A Preparation (eastern backhand grip).

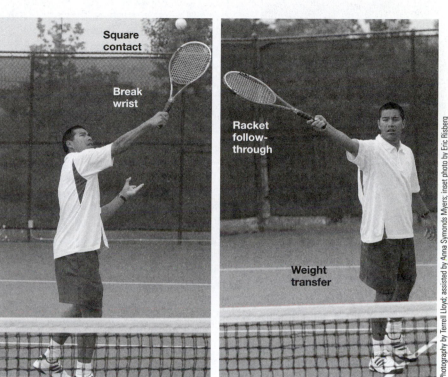

Photo 5.4B Contact.

Photo 5.4C Follow-through.

Photography by Terrell Lloyd; assisted by Anna Symonds Myers; inset photo by Eric Risberg

to adjust to the falling pattern of the ball.

Bouncing the overhead means permitting the ball to bounce before executing an overhead. In two situations the lob is allowed to bounce prior to being hit as an overhead. Lobs that have a very high loft are permitted to bounce for better timing when hitting the overhead. Lobs that are short at the net, eliminating a good set position for the overhead, also are allowed to bounce.

Hitting a high lob following a bounce is similar to hitting the overhead from a mid-air position following a lob. The additional time generated when permitting a bounce gives the opponent an opportunity to reposition in anticipation of returning an overhead return, and it also gives the player hitting the overhead a chance to place the ball more effectively.

When hitting a lob that bounces short, you need to stay low enough so the stroke is still angled down and through the ball. The goal for

the overhead return of a short ball is a short, hard-hit, high-bouncing ball that carries out beyond the baseline.

The *backhand overhead* (also called "high backhand volley") is used when the player cannot run around the ball to hit a forehand overhead. To begin a backhand overhead, the player should use an eastern backhand or continental grip and turn the shoulder so the racket side actually faces the net. The elbow on the racket side is up and points to the ball, and the racket head is below the hand. The weight is on the player's back foot and the head is up, eyes fixed on the ball.

The ball is contacted above the head slightly in front of the racket shoulder, with the racket face moving through the ball with a strong break of the wrist. The weight is transferred forward through the ball, with the follow-through carrying the racket head downward and parallel to the court surface (Photo 5.4A–C).

Incorporating the overhead into the total game blends favorably with the player's total game plan. The overhead is the second type of shot that is hit before the ball bounces, thus joining the volley shot as a stroke hit in the air near the net. When a player is at the net, the opponent must hit either a groundstroke that the net player hopefully can volley, or a lob that the net player can return as an overhead.

Players with improving skill and confidence can hit an overhead from any location on the court, while beginning players should hit overheads when lobs are short between the service court line and the net. Beginning players also would be wise to let the ball bounce before executing an overhead, so timing can aid in the stroke. As they develop skill, the transition to a complex overhead can be hitting on the fly and using the scissors kick.

Regardless of skill development, the player has to remember that the overhead is an offensive shot that must be hit under control and with confidence. The player also should remember that the overhead is the first in a series of overheads if the opponent returns the first overhead. Returns of overheads tend to be shorter lobs than the first lob hit, consequently setting up the player at the net for an eventually "easy" overhead.

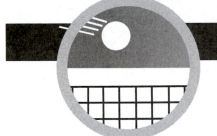

Points to Remember

Orthodox Forehand Overhead

1. Keep in mind that the forehand overhead is consistent with a basic throwing action that imitates the flat serve.
2. Place the racket head between your shoulder blades on the backswing.
3. Point your non-racket arm at the ball for a reference point to the ball.
4. Keep the base of the feet wide throughout the stroke.
5. Bring the racket through the ball with a wrist snap and a downward follow-through.
6. "Bounce" the ball when it is lobbed extremely high or is hit short to the net.

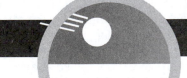

Points to Remember

Backhand Overhead

1. Point the racket elbow at the ball on the backhand overhead, and turn the racket side to the net during the preparation phase.
2. Bring the wrist through the ball forcefully on the backhand overhead.

Common Errors and How to Correct Them (Forehand Overhead)

The Error	What Causes the Error	To Correct the Error
Hitting into the net.	Ball too far out in front of the lead shoulder, or hitting the ball downward.	Get directly underneath the ball. Keep your chin up.
Hitting out beyond the opponent's baseline.	Hitting too hard with poor timing, or hitting up into the ball.	Get directly underneath the ball and hit through the ball, breaking at the wrist at contact.
Inconsistency in placing the ball.	Racket not placed between the shoulder blades on the backswing, and player's position under the ball is random.	Get directly underneath the ball, and always place the racket between the shoulder blades.
Hitting the ball off the edge of the racket at the top, or off the bottom edge, causing the ball to be hit long or to hit the court surface immediately.	Swinging too early or too late.	Point the non-racket arm to the ball for a reference point, check the position of the racket on the backswing, and develop a rhythmical timing to the stroke.

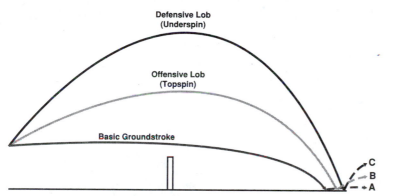

Figure 5.1 Flight patterns of lobs and groundstroke.

The Lob

The **lob** is an extension of the groundstroke, incorporating the same grip and basic swinging action. Mechanics of the stroke require the racket face to open and lift the ball up rather than hit through the ball. Lobs are characterized by a high *flight pattern* and can be both offensive and defensive. The flight patterns are different for each type of lob, and the differences are based on the purpose of the stroke and the amount of spin applied to the ball. The beginning player initially is simply trying to get the ball in the air, over the head of an opponent. In a short time span; however, the beginning player has to learn to hit two types of lobs. The two basic lobs used in tennis are discussed next and are diagrammed in Figure 5.1.

The *defensive lob* has a high flight pattern and is hit off a strong opposing-player return, with an underspin rotation. The *offensive lob* has a lower flight pattern than the defensive lob and is hit over the outstretched reach of the net player, bouncing near the baseline and kicking on beyond the baseline.

The *defensive lob* is the typical lob hit by beginning players. As they develop skills, beginners use the defensive lob as a reaction to an opponent's overhead. With an eastern forehand or backhand grip, the racket is brought back into a short backswing position with a firm wrist. The racket is brought forward to hit the ball off the lead shoulder. The bottom edge of the racket leads, opening the racket face. The

Defensive Lob with Forehand Underspin

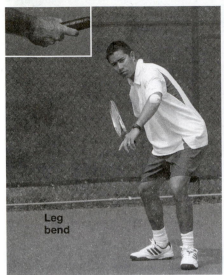
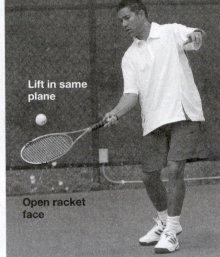
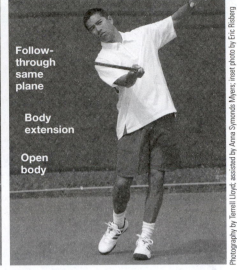

Photo 5.5A Preparation (eastern forehand grip).

Photo 5.5B Contact.

Photo 5.5C Follow-through.

Defensive Lob with Backhand Underspin

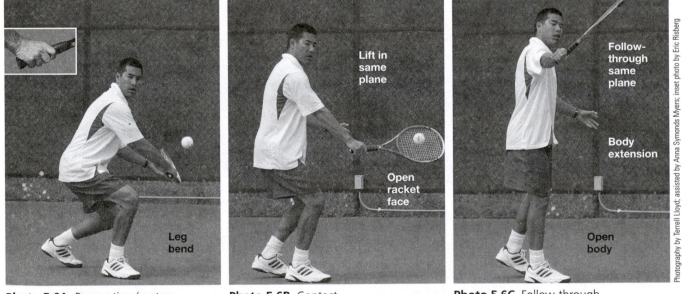

Photo 5.6A Preparation (eastern backhand grip).

Photo 5.6B Contact.

Photo 5.6C Follow-through.

follow-through is high, and the racket face remains open. The racket stays in the same plane as during the swing from preparation to contact. The wrist remains firm throughout the stroke, and the weight transfer, although important, is minimal compared to other strokes. The legs are bent and extended through the swing pattern, but only with a minimum amount of change. The lob is a reaction to an aggressively hit ball, so the total stroke has to be in moderation to combat the high velocity of the ball (Photos 5.5A–5.6C).

The *offensive lob* is really an extension of a topspin groundstroke

Forehand Offensive Lob with Topspin

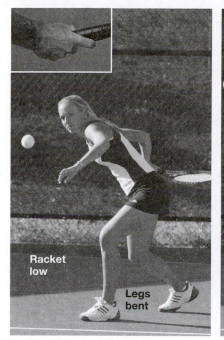

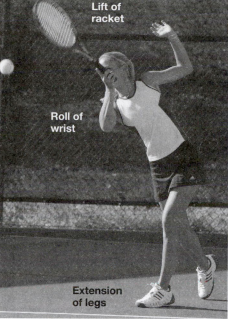

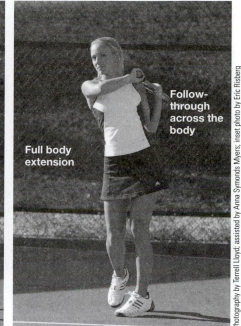

Photo 5.7A Prior to contact (eastern forehand grip).

Photo 5.7B Just after contact.

Photo 5.7C Follow-through.

described in Chapter 2 on page 27 for topspin forehand and page 28 for backhand groundstrokes. It requires use of an eastern forehand or backhand grip.

The racket is brought back low with an extensive knee bend and the wrist cocked. The racket then moves into the ball with a slightly open face at waist height, meeting the ball from underneath and lifting up. The wrist breaks at contact, imparting topspin to the ball. The follow-through continues with the racket finishing at an exaggerated high position off the middle of the body, with a roll of the wrist (Photos 5.7A–5.8C). The more speed generated by the racket head, the more topspin generated, and the faster the ball will drop.

Racket control, weight transfer, and movement of the feet are essential to hitting lobs. These skills require extensive work on the part of a beginning player. Racket control is used to apply topspin of varying degrees, underspin, or a simple block of the ball.

Weight transfer, as with all shots, is important with the lob, but the transfer has more to do with the hips and a little step transfer than with a long step into the ball. It is more of a center-of-gravity movement forward.

Most lobs are hit on the move rather than from a stationary position. The player either is retreating from the net to hit the ball or is moving laterally along the baseline. As a result of having to hit a lob on the run, the lob isn't always a nice setup from a ready position that permits easy execution of the stroke. Moving the feet to get to the ball, then recovering enough to place the racket on the ball while attempting to hold form, are all based on the initial foot movement and anticipation as to the location the opponent has intended for a target (Photos 5.9A–C and 5.10A–C).

Incorporating the lob into the total game is important to the developing player. Without the lob, there is no response to the overhead smash and the options for hitting

Backhand Offensive Lob with Topspin

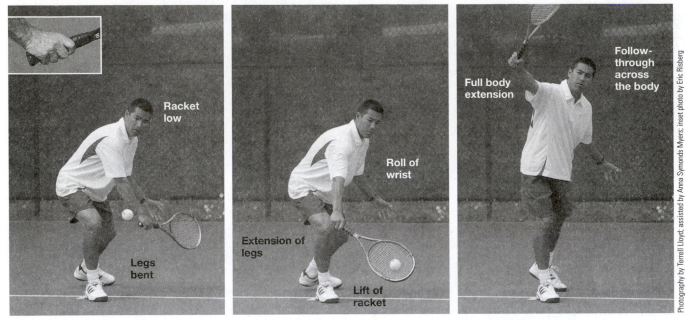

Photo 5.8A Preparation (eastern backhand grip).

Photo 5.8B Contact.

Photo 5.8C Follow-through.

Moving Laterally to Hit a Lob Behind the Baseline—Forehand

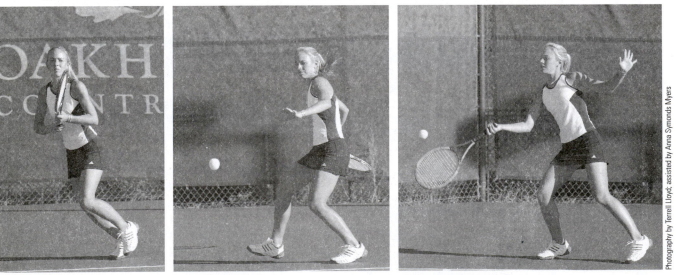

Photo 5.9A Preparation.

Photo 5.9B Backswing.

Photo 5.9C Contact.

a ball when the opponent is at the net decrease by one. The lob also serves as an occasional change-of-pace stroke, and it can be frustrating for the opponent who likes pace associated with the game or who cannot hit an overhead effectively. The lob is an extension of a ground-stroke, and developing the skill is a transition rather than development of a totally new stroke.

Retreating to Hit a Lob Behind the Baseline—Backhand

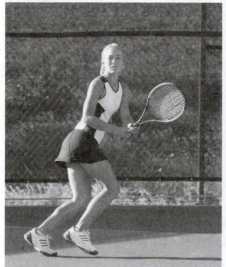
Photo 5.10A Preparation.

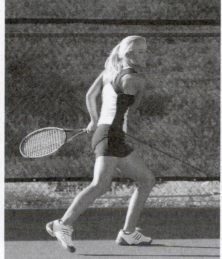
Photo 5.10B Backswing.

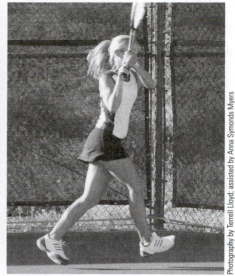
Photo 5.10C Follow-through.

Photography by Terrell Lloyd; assisted by Anna Symonds Myers

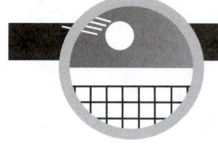

Points to Remember

Lobs

1. To produce an offensive lob with topspin, roll the forearm from contact through follow-through.

2. Strive for all lob follow-throughs to finish high.

3. Follow the principle that the more defensive a lob, and the more change from some topspin to an underspin, the more firm the wrist and shorter the backswing.

4. Follow through an underspin to a ball on the defensive lob in the same plane.

5. To regulate topspin in an offensive lob, vary leg bend and extension. The more topspin, the more leg bend and extension.

6. Open the racket face on lobs at contact.

7. Move to the ball as quickly as possible to incorporate form into the stroke.

Common Errors and How to Correct Them (Lobs)

The Error	What Causes the Error	To Correct the Error
Lobs hit long beyond the opponent's baseline.	Too much velocity and lift applied to the ball.	The lob requires touch and feel. Focus on a shorter target. Adjust the upward angle of the racket.
Balls hit short just over the net.	Usually not enough follow-through and backswing.	If stroking the lob, the backswing and follow-through should be equal in distance; and the more distance, the farther the ball will travel.
Lobs that are blocked rebound off at different angles.	Racket face isn't square to the ball.	Provide a firm arm and wrist base with an open racket face.

Checkpoints ✔✔

1. Positioning to hit an overhead smash requires the body to
   a. be positioned behind the ball.
   b. be positioned in front of the ball.
   c. be positioned underneath the ball.
   d. adjust depending on the height of the lob.

2. The overhead smash should be hit after allowing the ball to bounce when
   a. a lob is hit short at the net.
   b. a lob has a very high loft.
   c. situations in both *a* and *b* exist.
   d. the player is unsure of how to hit the ball.

3. When hitting a backhand overhead, the position of the elbow is
   a. up, pointed at the ball.
   b. out, pointed in line with where the ball is to be hit.
   c. down, positioned to allow the racket to swing through the ball.
   d. none of the above.

4. Overhead smash shots hit long are caused by
   a. hitting the ball too hard.
   b. hitting the ball with an open racket face.
   c. hitting the ball with the ball positioned behind the head.
   d. all three examples above.

5. When hitting an offensive lob, the follow-through pattern requires the racket
   a. to cross the upper body and finish high.
   b. to stay in the same plane as with the backswing and contact positions.
   c. to stop following contact with the ball.
   d. to cross the upper body and stay low.

6. The ball action off a defensive lob is
   a. underspin.
   b. topspin.
   c. slice.
   d. no spin.

7. The flight patterns of a basic groundstroke, offensive lob, and defensive lob are
   a. high, middle, low.
   b. middle, high, low.
   c. low, middle, high.
   d. middle, low, high.

8. The keys to hitting successful lobs include
   a. leg bend and extension, open racket face, and fast racket movement.
   b. leg bend and extension, open racket face, and high follow-through.
   c. leg bend and extension, closed racket face, and high follow-through.
   d. leg bend and extension, closed racket face, and fast racket movement.

Answers to Checkpoints can be found on page 147.

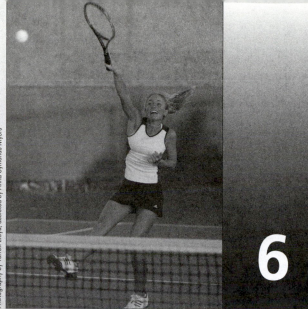

Photography by Terrell Lloyd; assisted by Anna Symonds Myers

6

Mental Aspects of Tennis Competition

At every level of tennis play, physical skill and mental strategy must be combined to be successful. Mental effort is the intangible that supports and reinforces the physical effort on a tennis court. Beginning tennis players tend to focus almost entirely on the physical aspect. Developing groundstrokes, volleys, serves, overheads, and lobs requires a tremendous concentration and effort. The early mental focus for a beginning tennis player is on how and where to hit a ball, and then on what the opponent is doing on the other side of the net. These are certainly important aspects in learning to play tennis, but a whole mental frame of mind is crucial to truly enjoying the game and to ultimately achieving success.

People play tennis for many reasons, including an interest and willingness to compete, a desire to play a social game, an interest in developing fitness, a way to gain college academic credit, or simply participating in an activity to add to quality of life. Whatever the reason for playing tennis might be, the most overriding should be the sheer joy of playing. To play tennis effectively requires that the player feel the game, feel the aesthetics, and appreciate the execution of skills related to the game. A successful tennis player plays for the enjoyment of physical movement and the fun that goes along with playing the game.

Tennis, as a game, includes sounds of ball striking racket, the wind, and the sounds a player makes when striving to hit a ball or move to the ball. Tennis is truly a life experience that can enhance the quality of life.

This chapter is about learning how to play tennis effectively. It is about gaining an understanding of what competition really means, eliminating negative thoughts and attitudes, developing the ability to concentrate and relax to reduce anxiety, and learning how to acquire mental toughness. The focus here is on playing tennis with a strong mental outlook. If you do that, all the other parts of the game, including winning, will fall into place.

67

Understanding What Competition Really Means

Competition and winning often are confused as being the same, but they are barely related. In competition, winning is a byproduct for one of the participants. Tennis competition does not pit opponent against opponent. It pits player against barrier. If you can visualize that the player on the other side of the net is setting up barriers, you are beginning to understand the nature of competition. The opponent—through a serve, a volley, or a lob—is creating a barrier for the other player to respond to. The barrier is erected for a challenge. It is nothing personal. To be successful in a match and learn to truly compete, a tennis player has to understand that concept.

A player must learn to emphasize *execution over winning*. If execution is the important aspect, the winning will take care of itself. Worrying about winning or losing interferes with execution and winning alike. Thinking about appearances or pleasing others interferes with execution and winning. The emphasis is on execution, the concentration is on execution, and the goal is execution.

When using the term "execution," a clarification is in order. The emphasis is not on thinking about executing a skill pattern; it is on completing the skill pattern. The mind should focus on feeling a barrier and responding to it by a reflex action, and that reflex action is execution. If a player begins to analyze movement and strokes, or begins to think of ulterior motives behind execution, skilled play collapses.

The beginning tennis player may not have been exposed to this concept before and so may have difficulty understanding why thinking about winning is not acceptable. If you can accept that emphasis on winning places pressure to excel and pressure not to fail, the idea of eliminating those pressures might become palatable. If executing by *doing* provides the realization of the long-term goal of winning, execution begins to make sense.

Eliminating Negative Attitudes

When participating in tennis, a *negative attitude* or *negative feelings* contribute to a negative response. If a player is ready to receive a serve and thinks, "Please don't make the serve; double fault—please," a negative attitude has been established. Other thoughts that are apt to enter the mind include, "What if I miss the shot?" or "If I hold my serve, I can win," or "You dummy—why can't you hit the ball?" Each of these plants a negative thought that contributes to a less than successful experience.

Negative attitudes arise when a player gets upset and begins to talk to the other self: "How could you hit such a stupid shot," or "I can't believe you're real—how could you miss such an easy setup?" If a player keeps making derogatory self-statements about performance, that player may well exceed all expectations of failure through negative thoughts.

Fear of winning and *fear of losing* both contribute to negative thought. Fear places pressure on the player not to make mistakes, and that negative thought reemphasizes fear of failure. The player becomes anxious to do well, and that anxiousness contributes to tension, which restricts performance, as performance must be accomplished in a relaxed, controlled manner.

Becoming *angry and losing one's temper* is another negative. Anger is a means of releasing energy, and this will take a toll on the player when a demand for extra effort is needed and the body cannot provide it. Losing one's temper also places pressure on that player. A player who gets mad at himself or herself is venting anger internally. That internal anger creates the same anxiety as the fear of winning or losing, with the player trying to please the self. The effect of the cycle of anger–anxiety-pressure is the collapse of the player's performance during competition.

Another negative associated with performance and tennis play is the opponent's behavior. A popular term in sport is "psych out." Behavior by an opponent can be upsetting if it is permitted to be upsetting. Body language, verbal comments, gamesmanship, and outbursts by an opponent can create negative reactions that will cause the other player to become anxious.

Negative thoughts can be changed by realizing what is happening and replacing them with positive thoughts. Instead of worrying about a missed shot, concentration should be on remembering a similar shot executed well. Instead of hoping that an opponent will miss a serve, a player should hope that the serve will be good so "I can have the opportunity to return a winner."

The fear of winning or losing is eliminated if the player will remember and practice what competition means and shut out the emphasis on winning and losing. Attacking one's own person verbally and sometimes physically is not being a friend to oneself. The developing player should treat the self with respect and dignity, stop arguing with and embarrassing the other self, and begin to compliment the other self on a good shot or a good point

played. The more *positive the self-talk*, the more potential for success. Positive self-talk, such as "Way to keep the ball deep on the baseline," "That's the way to hit with control," or "Keep pushing—I have her on the run" are examples of *positive self-talk*. Finally, not allowing an opponent to psych you out is extremely helpful in competition.

Concentration

Concentration is an important part of tennis. Blocking out all factors other than executing a shot is required for success. A focus on the ball and the task of hitting the ball helps a player to concentrate. When engaged in a rally, the player should look at the seams of the ball all the way to the racket face. Research indicates that a player can see a ball only to within 4 feet of the racket, and just the effort to look the ball into the racket improves concentration.

Concentration also is enhanced by being in touch with one's own body. The ability to synchronize breathing with each stroke and to sense the heartbeat as a body function permit the player to be in touch and concentrate better.

Another sense that enhances concentration is hearing—as in hearing the tennis ball make contact with the racket strings. And the kinesthetic sense is evoked when feeling the impact of ball and racket and recognizing muscle contraction and tension during the stroke. To really concentrate requires the player to eliminate all extraneous aspects of the environment.

Exchanging sides of the court can be a time for concentration. The concentration should be on the game plan and on thinking positive thoughts. If a player keeps saying, "I'm playing well," that thought will

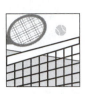

become reality. In sum, concentration means focusing on the task at hand.

Anxiety and Slumps

There will be times when everything "clicks" during a game—a *flow* to movement and to the play in general. That flow might last for a few points in a match, for a larger portion of a match, for a few days, or for months. Then there will be down times, when nothing seems to work. The down time is described best as a *slump*. Slumps seem to appear for no reason, but they usually result from worry, tension, or a fear of winning or losing.

In short, slumps occur as a result of self-induced pressure, and that pressure causes anxiety. Once a player becomes anxious, the muscles tense, which in turn forces physical errors because there is no relaxation during play. When the errors mount, the tension increases and the slump continues. As long as the player permits the pressure to interfere with performance, the cycle will continue.

The cure for the slump is to eliminate the anxiety by reducing muscle tension. This is done in two ways:

1. The player begins to think positive.

2. The player begins to relax and hit out on each ball, eliminating concern for the end result.

To reduce muscle tension, the player has to rebuild confidence. Participating in a match with a player who hits at a consistent pace is a start at redeveloping that confidence. Self-talk ("good shot—way to play") aids in raising self-confidence. Believing that the flow will return and relaxing are keys to coping positively. As a means of relaxing, the player must work at minimizing the number of times the muscle groups will be permitted to tense, which

lessens interference with relaxed performance.

During competition, the flow may disappear when the player realizes, "I shouldn't be playing this well." A self-fulfilling prophecy begins to make the player anxious, and the whole cycle within the match begins to develop. In the next match a slump may not be evident, but somewhere in the match, if similar circumstances arise, play will deteriorate just as before. Regardless of the duration of the slump, the anxiety produces muscle tension, which reduces performance.

Relaxation

The ability to relax contributes greatly to physical performance. Learning how to relax in a tennis match requires first recognizing muscle tension. If the player grips the racket too tightly (an exception is when hitting volley shots), the muscles tense too much. With a little practice, shoulder and arm muscles that are tight can be recognized. A check of the jaw will reveal tenseness in the mouth and jaw areas. The whole body can tense during the pressure of a point or game, and shortness of breath, excessive sweating, and mental confusion are signals that the stress is too great. Relaxation during play can be attained in several ways:

1. By immediately responding to tension on the court.

2. By preparing to play through mental rehearsal and mental imagery.

3. By relaxing before the match.

The *immediate response to tension on the court* is to learn how to recognize the tension and then relax those muscle groups. If the player feels tension in the shoulders and neck, a clockwise rotation of the head followed by a counter-clockwise motion will relax that area. Tension in the arms and legs can be eliminated by running or skipping in place. Another exercise that aids in total body relaxation is to take a deep breath and hold for a count of five, finally expelling the air.

Preparing to play by using *mental rehearsal* or *mental imagery* requires practice, but it can be learned in a short time. The idea is to prepare so well mentally that it enhances confidence, which, in turn, reduces anxiety and tension. Among the several approaches to this way of developing relaxation, a skill problem can be corrected by visualizing the mistake, then repeatedly reviewing the proper skill in the mind.

Sometimes the skill problem is related more to the sequence of shots or a game plan. The corresponding mental practice should be to use imagery emphasizing the acceptable shot or sequence of shots in a game plan. This mental imagery is a foundation for the actual tennis match and will assist the player in recognizing specific situations. Mental rehearsal even helps during a match when a player visualizes a positive picture of the next sequence of serves or a strategy for moving the ball from one side of the court to the other in a baseline rally.

The most widely used technique for *pre-match relaxation* is *progressive relaxation*. It involves developing a habitual 20-minute-per-day relaxation exercise plus a before-a-match session. Skill development centers on recognizing muscle tension followed by relaxing each muscle group. The tension recognition and relaxation response provides a foundation from which to approach life in general, and tennis, in a more relaxed way. This skill carries over to a tennis match by permitting the player to recognize pressure during play, and immediately relaxing enough to prevent deterioration of performance.

Other forms of relaxation include meditation and self-hypnosis, beneficial to tennis players who want to improve their performance. The progressive relaxation technique and additional forms of pre-match relaxation also contribute to the player's using mental rehearsal or imagery after attaining relaxation.

The mental aspect of tennis preparation can raise a player's skill to a level not considered possible. The game is more mental than physical. By applying various forms of relaxation, the player will improve rapidly.

Mental Toughness

Jim Loehr ("How to get Mentally Tough," Parts I and II, *Tennis*, July/August 1992, pp. 45–61) provides excellent insights into mental toughness and how to mentally prepare for a match. He uses terminology analogous to muscular strength—resilience, emotional strength, flexibility, and responsiveness—in his definition of mental toughness.

Resilience relates to any emotional excess baggage carried into the next point of a match following a mistake. If your skill errors come in bunches, you may struggle with your temper and develop a negative attitude. If a bad call upsets you, you are not a resilient tennis player. To overcome weak resilience, focus on the positive. Avoid drooping or whining after you miss a shot. Turn away from the net—and leave the mistake behind you.

Players with *emotional strength* generate positive emotional support for themselves and reject negative emotional distress. Those who lack emotional strength are shy about pumping a fist in the air or showing positive emotion, are fearful of looking an opponent in the eyes, make a line call softly, and rarely question obviously bad calls. Emotional strength is displayed on the court through body language, voice patterns, and general attitude. Opponents sense weak behavior and uncertainty. The keys are to assume a court presence: Stand up straight, move with a purpose, use a firm voice in your calls, and don't complain.

Flexible players create a relaxed atmosphere in stressful situations. Laughing at a stupid mistake, ignoring poor court conditions or an obnoxious opponent, avoiding tantrums, and looking and feeling positive under all circumstances are marks of a flexible player. Positive thoughts and actions are critical to flexibility.

Finally, a *responsive* player maintains alertness and intensity. Behaviors such as playing in a daze, being too casual, forgetting the score, and not caring contribute to an unresponsive attitude. A responsive player focuses on the event and maintains a standard of expectation for a high performance level.

A great deal of mental effort is involved when playing tennis. Understanding what competition really is, eliminating negative attitudes, and developing relaxation techniques are extremely helpful.

Putting It All Together

Beginners and more experienced players alike would do well to apply the suggestions discussed in the previous pages. Think a little about how you might be most effective against another player in terms of mental outlook.

1. Don't be intimidated by an opponent. You are playing a barrier, not an opponent. You need to be confident that you are going to play as well as you are capable of playing.

2. Establish a plan of attack. The next two chapters offer the opportunity to develop strategies to compete in singles and doubles play. Think through what you are going to do—make it a mental plan.

3. Once you have started playing, recall what has been going on during the match. What are the strengths of the other player? Just as important, what are the weaknesses? Take advantage of the weaknesses. Within your skill level, try to hit shots to the weakness of the other player, and try not to hit the ball to any of the player's strengths ("Mind over Matter," by J. F. Murray, *Tennis*, May 1999, p. 20).

Confidence breeds confidence. Believe in yourself and what you have learned as a player up to the point of the most recent match you have played. Focus on your task. Think about what you have to do. It helps to have a desire to play well, and to be mentally and emotionally ready. You also must focus on the *process*, not the result. Enjoy the moment. Hit each ball as if it is your best shot. Have fun. And play for the sheer joy of playing. Learn to play with low anxiety. Dismiss being nervous, relax your body without becoming a wet noodle, and believe that you can play the game ("Even the Odds," by J. Taylor, *Tennis*, November 1999, p. 15).

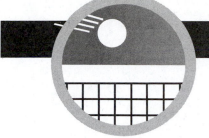

Points to Remember

The Mental Game

1. Competition is not opponent against opponent; it's player against barrier.
2. Emphasize execution over winning.
3. Eliminate negative attitudes including fear of losing, becoming angry, and self-defeating negative conversations with yourself.
4. Concentrate by blocking out extraneous interference.
5. Dispel anxiety.
6. Learn to relax on the court through relaxation techniques, including mental imagery and progressive relaxation.
7. Develop a mental toughness that includes resilience, emotional strength, flexibility, and responsiveness.
8. Establish a strong mental outlook, with confidence, match planning, and readiness.

Checkpoints ✔✔

1. Competition associated with tennis is most closely allied with
   a. winning.
   b. execution.
   c. thinking about execution.
   d. opponent against opponent.

2. Negative attitudes associated with tennis include all but one of the following:
   a. Anger
   b. Fear of winning
   c. Psyching out
   d. Shutting out emphasis on winning

3. Concentration associated with tennis includes all but one of the following:
   a. Focus
   b. Synchronized breathing
   c. Competing
   d. Hearing the tennis ball bounce

4. Slumps when playing tennis are caused by all but one of the following:
   a. Anxiety
   b. Flow
   c. Muscle tension
   d. Self-induced pressure

5. Relaxation during play can be attained by
   a. overcoming tension through will power.
   b. immediately responding to tension on the court.
   c. preparing to play through mental rehearsal.
   d. relaxing before the match.

6. A mentally tough tennis player meets all but one of the following profiles:
   a. Resilience
   b. Emotional strength
   c. Anxiousness
   d. Flexibility

7. Mental imagery requires
   a. emphasizing an acceptable shot.
   b. visualizing a positive picture of a skill sequence.
   c. visualizing a correction to a mistake.
   d. all of the above.

8. Muscle tension relates negatively to
   a. enhanced performance.
   b. failure to execute properly.
   c. focus on fundamentals.
   d. all of the above.

Answers to Checkpoints can be found on page 147.

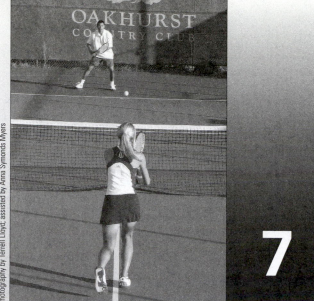

Photography by Terrell Lloyd; assisted by Anna Symonds Myers

7

Singles Strategy

Strategy in singles is part physical and part mental. The physical provides the mechanics to execute what the mental suggests be done to win a point. The mental is divided into two parts: (1) thinking and broadening thought to plan for the whole match, and (2) using the mind to control the match. This chapter is concerned with the physical or mechanical execution of what the mind suggests and requires in developing a game plan.

Percentage Tennis

Tennis is a game of mistakes. The player who makes the most mistakes loses. To win at tennis requires a system of play called **percentage tennis**. Percentage tennis is specific to hitting every ball deep and within the lines of the tennis court. This sounds easy, and actually it is, if you are devoted to the system of play. The problem with percentage tennis is that players would rather hit the one spectacular shot than play the ball methodically. A percentage player is one who plays within the

limits of skill, hitting only the shots that skill development will permit. In addition, the percentage player hits the appropriate stroke for a given shot. A percentage tennis player should grasp two concepts.

1. Comprehend what shot should be hit from what position on the court.

2. Understand and be able to apply the *division line theory of play*.

Court-Division-for-Position-Play Strategy

The tennis court is divided into three parts: backcourt, No Man's Land, and forecourt (Figure 7.1). The **backcourt** extends a yard deep behind the baseline, and this is where the percentage player returns all deeply hit shots from the opponent. The percentage concept requires that the player try to return every shot from the backcourt deep to the opponent's court.

The **forecourt** is between the service court line and the net. All shots in this area are volleys,

75

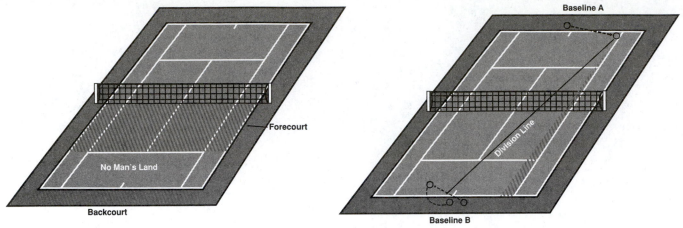

Figure 7.1 Court division for position play.

Figure 7.1 Court division for position play.

Figure 7.2 Division line theory of play.

overheads, or approach shots. This is the area the player should enjoy, because a ball hit in the forecourt represents an opponent's error and permits the percentage player to control the net area.

The **No Man's Land** is the portion of the court where the percentage player must step to return a shot, then retreat to the baseline to play the next shot. A player never should stand in this area. It is a highly vulnerable area and should be avoided.

Understanding and Applying Division-Line-Theory-of-Play Strategy

A second consideration in percentage tennis is to understand and apply the **division line theory of play**. This involves dividing the court into two equal parts on every stroke. If two players are rallying from the baseline and the ball is coming straight back to each player, the court is divided at the center mark on the baseline (Figure 7.2). If Baseline A player hits a ball angled to the left of Baseline B player, and then the return is a comparable cross-court return, a division line has to be established. This division line is established for Baseline B player by that player setting up on the baseline a step and a half to the left of the center mark. The intent is to maintain an equal court coverage

for a forehand or backhand return. The shaded area in Figure 7.2 helps illustrate this equal court balance.

If the percentage player can stay out of the No Man's Land except to return a shot, can apply the division line theory, and can hit each return deeply at least three times in a row, the percentage of the opposing player losing the point is quite high. When hitting from the baseline, the percentage player should use the increased skill shot of the topspin groundstroke when possible because of the high, safe trajectory and the deep, abrupt drop of the ball at the far baseline.

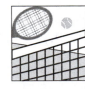

Service Strategy

Using the *service as a part of strategy* (Photo 7.1) is a necessity. Most beginners breathe a sigh of relief when their serve strikes the appropriate service court. The strategy comes into play when the serve strikes the service court because the server had confidence, hit the ball with velocity, and had a plan as to where to place the ball in the service court.

If a server can hit a serve repeatedly with modest speed and place the ball in the corners of the opponent's service court 70 percent of the time, the chances for success

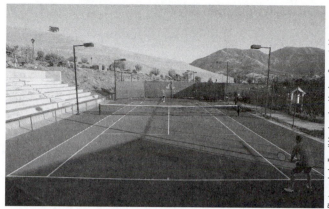

Photo 7.1 Service and service return position.

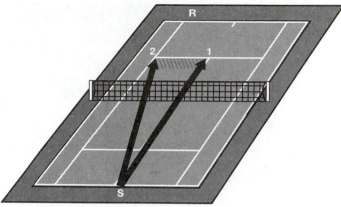

Figure 7.3 Hitting deep serves.

are enhanced greatly. If spin can be applied to the ball during service, with accuracy, a variety of serves can be used to confuse the receiver. In addition, the server can capitalize on the receiver's weakness in returning a serve if those weaknesses can be recognized.

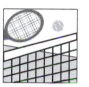

Return-of-Service Strategy

Return-of-service strategy is crucial. The server's role is to place the ball in play, and the return player's role is to keep the ball in play. The strategy is to hit the ball back with pace, and to hit it deep to eliminate the server's initial advantage. The server who relies on the serve to win points will begin to lose confidence if the ball keeps coming back.

Increasing Beginner Skills: Placement and Service Strategy

Placement of the service should be deep (Figure 7.3). Then choices can be made as to where to direct the ball to cause the most problems for the receiver. From a position of S1 (Figure 7.4) a serve may be hit down the center of either service court. From a position of S2, a serve is hit

wide to either service court. These placements are excellent spots to place a service. In addition, if a server puts reasonable velocity on a flat serve, the receiver will have problems even if the ball is placed directly in front of the body.

A more advanced slice serve can be hit wide to the right side of the right service court, pulling the receiver off the court and consequently opening the whole court for the next shot by the server (Figure 7.5). A slice service to the right corner of the left service court pulls the receiver to the middle of the court, causing a down-the-middle return (Figure 7.6).

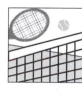

Increasing Beginner Skills: Second-Service Strategy

The second service is even more important in the sense that if it is not placed accurately in the appropriate service court, the point is lost without a response from the receiver. The second serve not only must be reliable and accurate but also should have some pace. Many servers make the mistake of pushing the ball into the service court rather than hitting with good form.

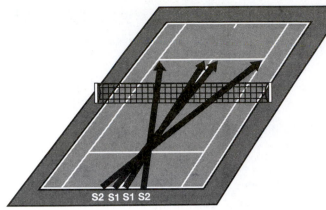

Figure 7.4 Hitting the corners on the serve.

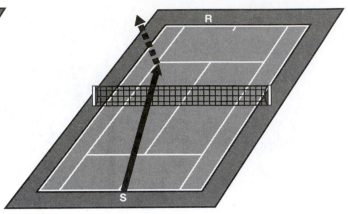

Figure 7.5 Placing slice serve.

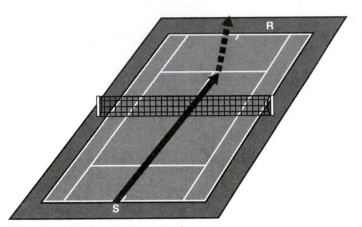

Figure 7.6 Placing slice serve to the left service court.

The three requirements of a sound second serve are:

1. The serve must have accuracy coupled with pace.

2. The serve must have spin to ensure accuracy.

3. The serve never is pushed or blooped into the service court. Accuracy is enhanced by a slice or service with some attention to placement of the ball and pace.

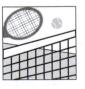

Increasing Beginner Skills: Return-of-Service Strategy

Once the beginner gains enough skill to get the ball back to the server, it is time to establish an expanded strategy. A cause–effect relationship indicates that the receiver should respond to the server's pace and depth of serve by standing beyond the baseline to return serve. This thought must be dispelled. If the server has a strong spin, it is best to step inside the baseline and cut down the sidespin or high bounce before the effect can occur. A serve that is pushed over the net should be returned firmly and deeply, and the receiver should avoid the tendency to "kill" the ball.

When returning the serve, the receiver can use various placements that will enhance the play at that point. Returning *down the line* is usually a mistake when the server has the ability and court position to move easily down the baseline to reach the ball, as it will leave the court open for a cross-court winner by the server (Figure 7.7).

Service returns are most effective when hit back along the line of flight of the serve and at the feet of the server. When serves are hit with little pace, the receiver has more options, including down the line, cross-court, and angled cross-court. The effort off a weak serve should be to hit a winner under control, forcing the opposing server to hit while moving to the ball, or to miss the ball entirely.

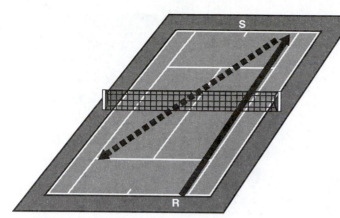

Figure 7.7 Consequences of return of serve down the line.

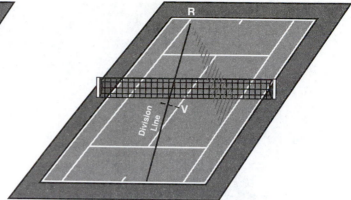

Figure 7.8 Division line theory.

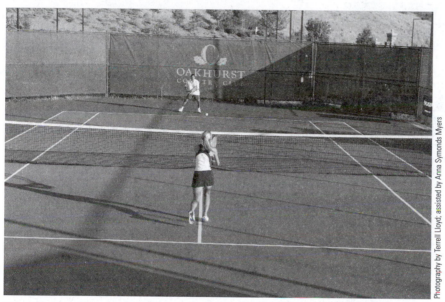

Photo 7.2 Server going to the net.

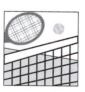

Increasing Beginner Skills: Attacking the Net and Beating the Net Player

Judgments a player must make include when to go to the net and, once there, when to stay and when to leave. A player should go to the net in three situations:

1. Off a serve.

2. Off an approach shot.

3. Off a firmly hit groundstroke that forces the opponent to

move behind the baseline when returning the shot.

When at the net, there are two times to stay and continue play at the net:

1. When following one volley with another.

2. When hitting an overhead from between the service court line and the net.

The player should retreat in only one situation: when a lob is hit deep to the baseline, compelling the net player to leave the net to return the lob. The player attacking the net should apply the *division line theory* by following the path of the ball to the net, dividing the court in half between the two players.

The division line will enable the net player to cover all territory equally between the forehand and the backhand and give the opponent only one possible winning shot. If, as an example, the net player hits to the opponent's deep, right baseline corner and takes a step and a half to the left of the center of the net, the only possible return for a winning shot is to the far right corner angled at the net (Figure 7.8).

Going-to-the-Net Strategy

Going to the net following a serve suggests the execution of an accurate serve (Photo 7.2). In fact, an

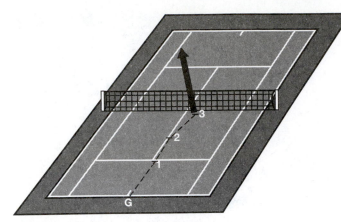

Figure 7.9 Going to the net following a serve.

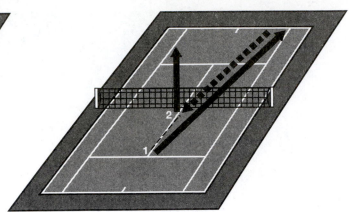

Figure 7.10 Going to the net following an approach shot from the middle of the court.

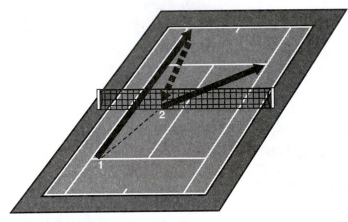

Figure 7.11 Going to the net following an approach shot from the sideline area of the court.

accurate serve with pace provides the opportunity to effectively advance to the net. If the serve is returned with pace, penetration is as close as it is going to be if the server can get to the service court line (Figure 7.9, Position 1). If the return of the serve is a mis-hit, the server can pounce on the return with an efficient volley from the net position (Figure 7.9, Position 2 or 3). If the return of serve is at the feet of the server, who has advanced on the net, a 20-foot return distance from the net may become a liability. The server now has to be an exceptional volleyer because the ball at the feet creates vulnerability. A slice service permits the server to advance closer to the net before being forced to stop and respond to the opponent's return of serve.

Going to the net following an approach shot is an ideal time to advance on the net (Figure 7.10).

If the return from the opponent is short—at the service line in the middle of the court—the approach shot can be played to a corner (Figure 7.10, Position 1). Once the ball is hit to the corner, the player advances to the net, in line with the ball, and volleys cross-court (Figure 7.10, Position 2). If a return shot is hit to the service line, close to and parallel to a sideline, the approach shot should be down the sideline (Figure 7.11, Position 1) followed by a short, angled volley cross-court as the player advances on to the net (Figure 7.11, Position 2).

Going to the net off a groundstroke must be done with some prudence. It is inadvisable to go to the net when the groundstroke

1. has not been hit with authority,

2. has not been hit deep to the baseline, or

3. has not forced the opponent to return the shot while moving away from the net.

If the player has hit an effective groundstroke, however, that player must learn to *close in on the net.* As the player advances to the net from the baseline, he or she must assume a ready position prior to the return shot crossing the net. Once the advancing player has hit a return, that player continues on to the net in a line with the ball, and again stops in

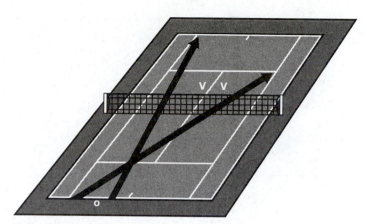

Figure 7.12 Hitting a passing shot to beat a net player.

a ready position before the return shot crosses the net.

Between two and three stops are required to gain control of the net and to be in control of hitting a winning shot if the opponent is able to respond with some authority in returning the shots hit by the advancing player. Three thoughts should be on the mind of the player advancing from the baseline:

1. Volley and advance.

2. Punch the ball deep to the baseline.

3. Hit at the feet of the opponent so the return is "up."

Advancing to the net is an adventure and a reward if the end result is a winning shot. The choice of going to the net is based on the advantage that it will give the player to advance. Some final thoughts associated with attacking the net are:

1. The volleyer always must stop and assume a ready position prior to the return shot crossing the net.

2. When attacking, the player should follow the path of the ball to provide the division line.

3. The player has to get close to the net to hit a volley. A beginning player needs to be a racket-and-a-half length away from the net, whereas a skilled player can

volley from the service court line. All players who volley must remember to stay low and punch the ball.

Beating-the-Net-Player Strategy

A *threefold strategy to beat the player who attacks the net* is to: (1) hit at the feet of the net player, (2) hit a passing shot, and (3) hit a lob.

Hitting at the feet of the net player forces the player to hit the ball up in the air, providing a setup to hit a winning return. Two shots are most often used to hit at the feet of a player at the net. A topspin stroke usually is hit from the baseline to the feet of a player at the net; and from a return of serve a ball often is blocked back to the feet of an advancing net player.

Hitting a passing shot to beat a net player is a second means of defeating the volleyer at the net. The passing shot may be hit down the line or as a short-angled cross-court shot. As an example, if a player is to the left of the center mark at the baseline, a shot down the net player's right sideline could pass that player. A ball hit farther to the left of the baseline player can be played as a short-angled cross-court passing shot, as the net player has moved to the right of center to establish the division line (Figure 7.12).

The third method of *beating the net player is with a lob.* A net player tends to get too close to the net to avoid hitting balls at the feet. This diminishes the ability to retreat and cover a deep lob, and the player at the baseline has a clear-cut choice of hitting an offensive, topspin lob to the net player's baseline. If the players are beginners, any form of a lob that gets over the head of the net player will be effective. The important point is to drive the opponent back from the net, ensuring a return on the move with the back to the net.

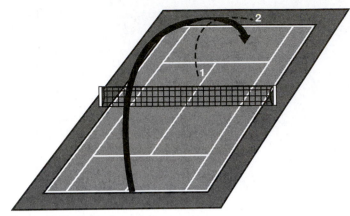

Figure 7.13 Retrieving a lob.

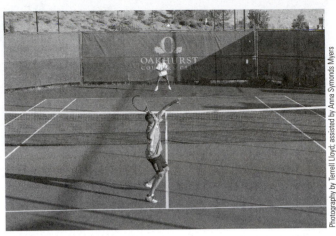

Photography by Terrell Lloyd; assisted by Anna Symonds Myers

Photo 7.3 Overhead set up.

Increasing Beginner Skills: Lob and Overhead Strategy

Lobs and overheads are an integral part of overall court strategy. The lob can be either a defensive or an offensive shot, and the overhead is a reward for effective serve or groundstroke play.

Lob Strategy

The questions in singles play are *when to hit a lob* and *what kind to hit.* Defensive lobs should be hit whenever the opponent has forced the play and whenever a player needs to "buy time" to recover from a strong shot. The important part of a defensive lob is to hit to the opponent's backhand, forcing the opponent to run around the ball to hit an overhead, or to return the ball going away from the net with a backhand stroke.

When retrieving a lob, the player, instead of running in a straight line, should run to the outside of the ball and come from behind it to hit a return lob, or a forceful groundstroke, or an overhead (Figure 7.13, Positions 1 and 2). A lob that has the effect of an offensive shot should, of course, be hit when the opposing net player is too close to the net.

Overhead Strategy

Overheads are used in singles strategy to respond to lobs that are hit between the service court and the net (Photo 7.3). Setting up is an important part of that strategy. A crisp volley down the opponent's right sideline forces that player to execute a lob that travels to the middle of the court, which, in turn, can be hit as an overhead to the opponent's left corner (Figure 7.14). This example illustrates that a firm offensive shot creates a weak lob return, and for each lob return there is a wide variety of targets for the overhead. Balls hit deep to the opponent's baseline always are acceptable as effective overheads (Figure 7.15).

When the return lob is closer to the net, overheads can be angled and bounced out of the opponent's court. The angle and bounce carry the ball into a nonreturnable location (Figure 7.16). Angled and deeply angled overheads are also effective (Figure 7.17). They ensure that the opponent has to move to retrieve the overhead rather than remain stationary and hit a lob with control. An angled overhead (Figure 7.17, Position 1) is an excellent placement for a backhand overhead because

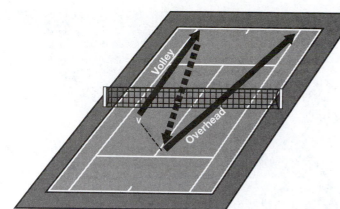

Figure 7.14 Setting up an overhead return with a volley shot.

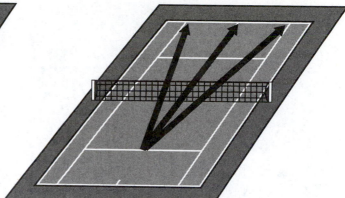

Figure 7.15 Hitting overheads deep.

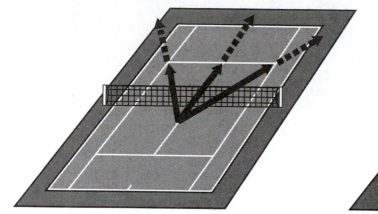

Figure 7.16 Hitting angled overheads.

Figure 7.17 Angled and deeply angled overheads.

accuracy in placement is more important than speed in completing the shot successfully, while a forehand overhead angled deep is often a winning shot (Figure 7.17, Position 2).

Often the first overhead is not a winning shot, nor should it be expected to be. The first overhead "softens up" the opponent, who can return the shot only from a defensive position. Strategically, if the player hitting the lob keeps the overhead consistently deep and angled, the opponent returning lobs eventually wears down or breaks down skill-wise and hits a short lob that can be returned as a winning overhead.

groundstrokes deep and relying on percentage tennis to its fullest. The idea is to force the opponent to make a mistake with a mis-hit shot or poorly hit return. Among the several ways of forcing an error from the opponent are cross-court and down-the-line shots (Photo 7.4).

Duplicating-the-Opponent's-Groundstroke-Return Strategy

Duplicating the opponent's return is good strategy because it puts pressure on the opponent to change the direction of the ball. Singles strategy dictates that if the opponent hits cross-court, the return should be cross-court until the opponent hits down the line. At that point, the player hitting has the option of returning in duplication down the line or coming back cross-court. In either case, the advantage is with

Increasing Beginner Skills: Baseline-Play Strategy

Baseline play involves giving complete, undivided attention to hitting

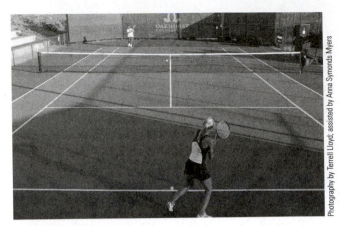

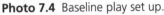

Photo 7.4 Baseline play set up.

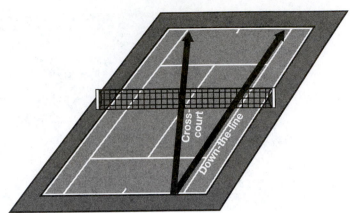

Figure 7.18 Duplicating groundstroke returns.

the player returning a shot rather than the opponent because the return angle favors the return player's stroke and because there is an element of the unknown in the return direction (Figure 7.18).

Moving-the-Opponent Strategy

Another strategy is to move the opponent back and forth across the baseline, forcing alternate forehand and backhand returns. If the opponent can be driven from one side of the court to the other, reaching for shot returns, the ball eventually will be returned short or "up" so an approach shot, volley, or overhead can be used as a follow-up to good baseline play.

With skill and experience, the baseline player can develop strategy using varied strokes, always coming back to hit with depth and angle that will cause the opponent to make a mistake. Sometimes varying the stroke is disguised by hitting down the sideline with a groundstroke to the opponent's backhand for a succession of shots, then switching to a cross-court shot that pulls the opponent out of a groove and requires a totally new stroke in the rally. Hitting the groundstroke again and again to the same side also will wear down an opponent's confidence, and the skill of the stroke will weaken as belief in winning the point lessens.

Scoring-Situation Strategy

Certain *scoring situations* in a match are vital to good strategy and success. In a game, a score of 30–15 is important because winning the next point will produce a score of 40–15. The leading player can use the 2-point difference as a lever to win the game within the next two points. If the 30–15 score becomes 30–30, either player may win the next two points.

A set score of 5–3 with the opponent serving is a crucial situation in the ninth game. If the opponent wins that game, the set is over at a 6–3 score. If the receiver of serve wins the ninth game, the score becomes 4–5 and the player who is behind serves with a tie set possible at 5–5 in the tenth game. Obviously, the 4–5 set score also is important, but the player behind is serving, and with a degree of serving skill, the server has the advantage. Other scores that are meaningful are the first point of any given game and the last point of a game, set, or match.

Game-Plan Strategy

The *overall game strategy and plan* are only as good as the player's skill. The game plan for an early beginner is to do the best possible to return shots back across the net. By the time the player can hit with some consistency, percentage tennis becomes really important. It means the advanced beginner can work at hitting the ball back with depth and patience and begin to set up an opponent with subtle techniques to force an error.

Continual maturation permits the player to understand that the mind is the most important part of the game. The ability to out-think the opponent becomes the key to victory. Changing pace, moving a player along the baseline, and moving the opponent to the net and back away from the net all begin to make sense.

The game plan and strategy for a player starts with the warm-up and ends with the last point of the match. In the warm-up, the player begins to assess the opponent's ability, being careful not to become overly confident of or intimidated by the opponent. During the warm-up, each player should determine the skills of the opponent and what strokes that opponent is capable of hitting effectively. The player who is assessing the other player should not change the game plan only to meet the opponent's skills, though. The assessing player must be able to react normally and not play as the opponent dictates.

As an example of a game plan: If the opponent likes to serve and volley, the strategy might be to prepare to hit passing shots, lobs, and groundstrokes at the opponent's feet. Another example is to stay at homebase during a rally and force the opponent to rally from the baseline when the opponent lacks consistency in hitting groundstrokes. Game plans and strategy should be a combination of the player reacting to the opponent's weaknesses and playing to the player's skill level.

Final game strategy thoughts are to:

1. Play every point and return every shot.
2. Look for the short ball, attack with an aggressive approach shot, and complete the attack by continuing on to the net.
3. Be consistent in play rather than hit the one spectacular shot.
4. Use defensive lobs to "buy time," as most tennis players cannot hit solid overheads in reacting to a lob.
5. Keep groundstrokes in play and deep.
6. Hit serves with pace and accuracy.

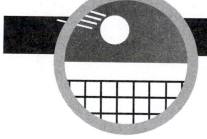

Points to Remember

Singles Strategy

1. Focus on playing *percentage tennis*.
2. Apply the *division line theory of play*, which, simply stated, is a division of a tennis court into two equal parts.
3. Effective placement of serve requires hitting down the center, wide, or directly at a receiver's body using both pace and spin.
4. Effective second-serve placement requires accuracy with pace—no blooping the serve.
5. Return serves should be deep and back, in line with the server's position.
6. Attack at the net after an effective serve, an approach shot, or off a firmly hit groundstroke that moves the opposing player.
7. Beat the net player by hitting at the feet, or hitting a passing shot, or hitting a lob.
8. Keep in mind that a game score of 30–15, and a set score of 4–5 are critical situations during a match.

Checkpoints ✔✔

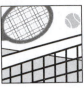

1. Percentage tennis is considered to be
   a. representative of who loses the most points.
   b. representative of who wins the most points.
   c. a strategy established to stay close in a match.
   d. none of the above.

2. The No Man's Land area is a non-official term used to describe
   a. a highly vulnerable area for a player to stand.
   b. another term for the service court area.
   c. the baseline area.
   d. none of the above.

3. The *division theory of play* means
   a. dividing the court into four parts.
   b. dividing the court into two equal parts.
   c. dividing the strategy of play into two parts.
   d. all three of the above.

4. In successful offensive service placement
   a. 50% of all serves must be "in."
   b. 70% of all serves must be hit into the deep corners of the opponent's service court.
   c. serves must be no less than 60% accurate.
   d. serves must be 80% accurate on a second serve.

5. Service returns are most effective when hit
   a. along the line of flight of the serve.
   b. down-the-line.
   c. along the line of flight of the serve at the feet of the server.
   d. cross-court.

6. It is inadvisable to go to the net when
   a. a groundstroke has been returned with no authority.
   b. a ball has not been returned deeply to the opponent.
   c. the opponent has not been forced to move away from the net.
   d. any of the above.

7. The three ways to beat a player at the net are to
   a. hit at the player's feet, pass the player, or lob.
   b. hit at the player, pass the player, or lob.
   c. lob, lob, and lob.
   d. rush the player at the net, pass the player, or lob.

8. Defensive lobs should be hit
   a. to attack the opponent's weakness.
   b. to "buy time."
   c. whenever the opposing player is aggressive.
   d. rarely since they are basically limited in success.

Answers to Checkpoints can be found on page 147.

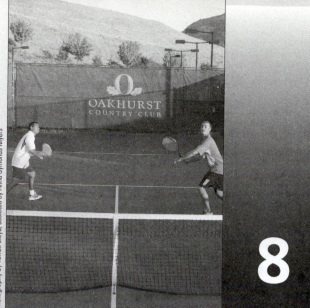

Photography by Terrell Lloyd; assisted by Anna Symonds Myers

8

Doubles Strategy

With the exception of the strokes used, doubles strategy is entirely different from singles strategy. Doubles is an attacking game, whereas singles tends to be a more passive defensive game. Doubles play is concentrated at the net or retreating from the net, whereas singles play is positioned at the baseline. The attacking concept of doubles provides an exciting type of match with quickly executed shots and good reactions. The beginner seldom experiences the challenge of doubles, yet this is the first situation a beginner may face if being taught in an instructional group.

Basic Alignments and Formations

Numerous formations are found in doubles play, including club or recreational social doubles (usually college-class doubles), conventional doubles, and mixed doubles. Choosing a partner and deciding where each partner will be aligned on the court is the beginning of a successful strategy.

Social Doubles

Beginning players should start from one of two formations, depending on how advanced the players are in executing strokes. These formations are associated with **social doubles**.

Two-Back Formation If the players have yet to be introduced to net play, including volleying and overhead smashes, it is best to begin doubles at the baseline in a *two-back formation* (Photo 8.1). The two-back formation also is used by experienced players when the opposing team is at the net hitting overheads while the two on the baseline team attempt to return lobs to defend against the overheads.

The weakness of the two-back formation is the defensive stature of the team and the lack of control at the net. A team that controls the net has an open court that allows large areas in which to place the ball for winning shots. From the baseline,

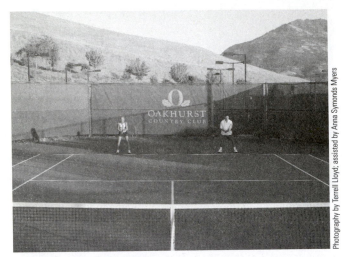

Photo by Terrell Lloyd; assisted by Anna Symonds Myers

Photo 8.1 Two-back formation.

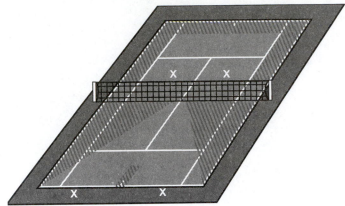

Figure 8.1 Target areas for two-up versus two-back.

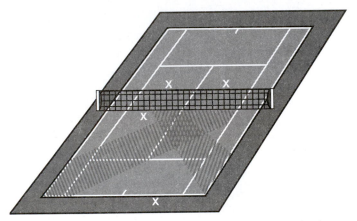

Figure 8.2 Target areas for two-up against one-up, one-back.

shots hit at players controlling the net have little potential for success because they involve only small target areas that the two players cannot cover at the net (Figure 8.1).

One-Up, One-Back Formation A second social doubles formation is *one up and one back*. This alignment is used when the players' experience at the net is at least adequate for protection at the net and for execution of firmly hit volleys.

One player up and one player back stems from the original alignment of the players in the serving and receiving positions. The problem arises when the server doesn't have the confidence to serve and follow the serve to the net or the return player does not follow the

return to the net. Once the alignment holds at one-up, one-back, that alignment becomes vulnerable to open-area winning shots. (See Figure 8.2 and Photos 8.2 and 8.3.)

Conventional Doubles: Two-Up in Tandem

Conventional doubles requires that a team attack the net and, if need be, attack face to face with the opposing team. The key to good doubles play is to work together in tandem. If the ball is lobbed deep when the team is at the net, the two must retreat together, and when one player hits an overhead from the service court line, they both must advance to the net together. Playing conventional doubles means working as a team, knowing where the other player is located, and depending on the partner to hit the appropriate shot. When controlling the net, the doubles team attacks side by side, positioned in the middle of the two service courts. From that position, as if they were on a string, the pair moves up and back and side to side in a balanced position (Photo 8.4).

A conventional formation can produce a significant number of movement patterns on the court. First, a teammate may *poach* in doubles. The definition is important. The poach means hitting a winning

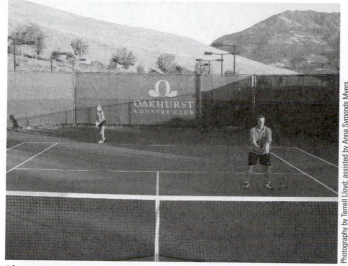

Photography by Terrell Lloyd; assisted by Anna Symonds Myers

Photo 8.2 One-up, one-back formation (serving).

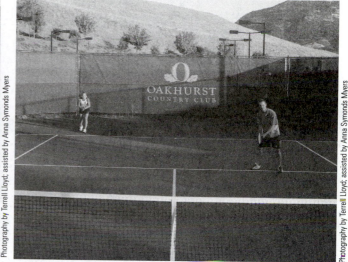

Photography by Terrell Lloyd; assisted by Anna Symonds Myers

Photo 8.3 One-up, one-back formation (receiving).

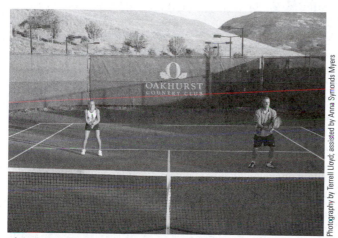

Photography by Terrell Lloyd; assisted by Anna Symonds Myers

Photo 8.4 Two-up formation (conventional doubles).

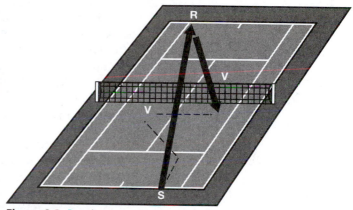

Figure 8.3 Poach movement patterns.

volley; it allows no margin for error. When poaching, the best target tends to be a volley directed at the feet of the net player. The net player steps across parallel to the net to hit a volley directed toward the partner at the baseline following a serve. The serving partner sees the poach attempt and veers to replace the position vacated by the poaching partner (Figure 8.3).

Another team movement pattern is to retreat to hit a lob, then recover for the next shot. The retreat incorporates a cross-action by team members to reach the ball. If the lob is to the deep left corner of the baseline, the partner on the right can see the ball and react to it better than the partner who would have to retreat in a straight line with the back to the opponents. At this point, the partners are at the baseline, where they will remain in a defensive posture until they can regain an advantage and return to the net (Photo 8.5 and Figure 8.4).

Mixed Doubles

Mixed doubles combines one male and one female partner. The formation is the same as for conventional doubles. The only real change is related to the physical strength and

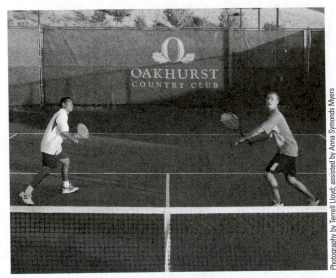

Photo 8.5 Retreat to return a lob (cross-action).

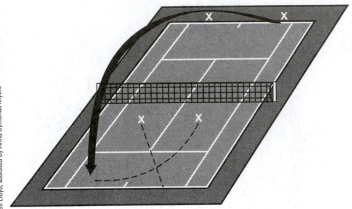

Figure 8.4 Movement pattern for retreating to return a lob.

skill of the female partner. If there is a strength and skill difference (the differences also could be between two male or two female partners), the alignment may have to be adjusted.

In playing mixed doubles, the opposing team typically attacks the female as often as possible. Therefore, when a female player serves to a female opponent, the male at the net must poach whenever possible. With the female serving, the server's velocity or pace usually is not as fast as when the male partner serves; consequently, the female server must stay in an up-back alignment. That alignment already has been identified as a weak formation, and it is the reason for the male partner's poaching. A serve to the backhand of the return player will aid the serving team by making it easier for the male partner to poach, and easier for the female partner to respond to a groundstroke return.

When receiving against the female server, one response might be a direct return back to the male net player. If successful, the male partner eventually will retreat to the baseline to avoid being hit by a return of serve.

A second strategy is to return serve cross-court. This subjects the server to returning a groundstroke

from a defensive position, and it avoids the male partner at the net.

Mixed doubles is a delightful game, and it can be highly competitive. Each partner has a role to play and a responsibility to fulfill. Strategy for mixed doubles can be enlarged to cover any doubles in which the characteristics are similar. If one partner is a physically stronger partner but the players are of the same sex, the same approach to strategy should be used.

Special Formations

Variations of formations can help a team in special situations. Two of these are Australian doubles and the I-formation.

Australian Doubles

Australian doubles eliminates an opposing team's cross-court return. In this alignment the server and net player are situated in a perpendicular line to the net with both players on the same side of the server's court. If the server is serving to the opposing team's right service court, the server will be to the right of the center mark and the net partner will be set up on the inside center of the serving team's right service court (Photo 8.6). This alignment leaves

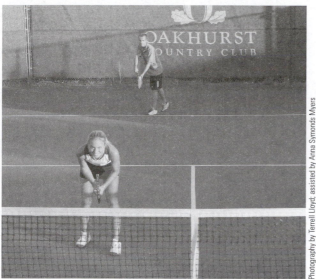

Photography by Terrell Lloyd; assisted by Anna Symonds Myers

Photo 8.6 Australian doubles formation.

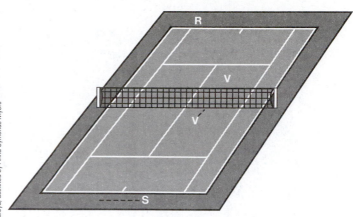

Figure 8.5 Movement pattern for Australian doubles formation.

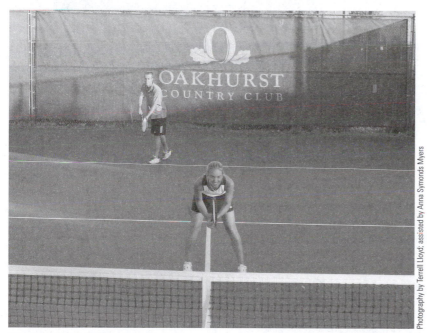

Photography by Terrell Lloyd; assisted by Anna Symonds Myers

Photo 8.7 I-formation.

the left service court of the serving team open during the serve. Following the serve, the baseline server moves to the left to cover the open court from the baseline. The partner at the net stays to create an up–back situation (Figure 8.5).

The Australian formation gives players several options. The first is for the net player to cross to the left service court following the serve while the serving partner moves farther to the right side of the baseline to protect that side of the court. A second option is for the team to crisscross following the serve, with the net player moving to the left and the server going straight to the net from the right side. A variation of the crisscross is for the server to follow the serve to the net on the left side, with the net player staying in the same position.

The more variations the Australian doubles formation can offer to the opposing team, the more confused those players will become. This formation is ideal for a team with one weak serving partner or a team with one partner who has a major skill weakness that this alignment can hide. Since the doubles alignment is strong down the middle of the court, it is important for the receiving team to return serve down-the-line.

I-Formation

Another special service formation is the I-formation (Photo 8.7). It positions the net player at the net, straddling the middle service court line. Its strength is down the middle, and if the server serves wide, forcing a cross-court return, the net player is positioned to respond with a potential winning volley. Actually, any serve that forces a return down the middle is advantageous to the

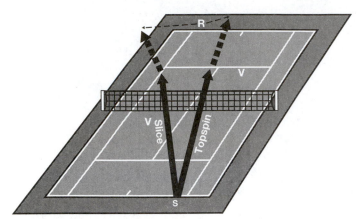

Figure 8.6 First-serve targets.

doubles serving team, but it also has a vulnerability that permits the receiving team to hit shots down the lines for winners.

The I-formation gives the receiving team a look that is different from the serving team and forces the opposing team to make adjustments. Sometimes even a small adjustment creates mistakes by the team that is doing the adjusting and works to the advantage of the more creative I-formation team. Response to the I-formation by the receiving team is consistent with response to the Australian doubles formation. That is, the target for return of serve should be down-the-line.

Service and Return-of-Service Strategy

Doubles play strategy is based on effective service and return of service. In addition, players can fully enjoy doubles play when they are consistent in executing serves and returning service.

Service Strategy

The first service in doubles is extremely important. Three-fourths of all first serves should be hit successfully to give the serving team the leverage of moving to the net as a team in a two-up volley situation. Once the developing player has progressed beyond hitting flat services with pace to areas of the opponent's service courts, spin serves should be used in most situations.

A slice serve can be effective when serving to the opposing team's right service court, to force the receiver off the court and to allow the attacking serving team to overplay to the left to control the net. Another effective serve, once a topspin serve has been developed, is a serve placement into the deuce service court inside corner. To reiterate, the service must be consistently accurate, and the placement, with spin, must be thoughtfully considered (Figure 8.6).

In addition, the beginner must work hard at protecting the partner at the net during service. A soft, pushed serve will endanger that partner and compel the team to play two-back on the serve, thereby defeating the advantage of the serving team in controlling the net.

Return-of-Service Strategy

Two considerations are attached to a *return of service* in doubles:

1. Get the ball back over the net at the serving team's feet.

2. Select the best target placement of the return, and then complete that task.

The first consideration is an obvious strategy related to self-preservation. The second consideration requires more planning and assessment of at least four options for target areas (Figure 8.7):

1. Return the ball to the feet of the net player or the advancing server.

2. Pass the net player.

3. Lob the net player.

4. Hit cross-court angled toward the server.

The first three options were discussed with singles strategy as they

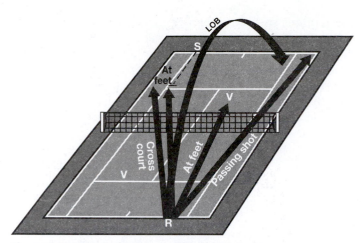

Figure 8.7 Options for return of service in doubles.

The best choice is a return at the attacking server's feet. A serve placement to the inside of the ad service court has the same response as the serve to the inside corner of the deuce service court. Serves hit wide to the respective service courts permit all four service return options to be used.

A major lesson to be learned is that a good server will give the receiver only a limited number of options from which to select during any given service situation. If a serve is well placed, the receiver will return serve to anticipated areas on the serving team's side of the court.

One last consideration of return of serve is for the receiving player to always get the racket on the ball. All strategy for a return of serve collapses if the receiver misses the return.

relate to playing a net player. With a service return, lobbing becomes difficult with a serve of any pace, but it is reasonably effective off a soft serve. If the net player does not advance on the net to within two steps from net position, the return at the net player can be effective also.

Passing the net player requires that the player at the net lean to the middle in anticipation of poaching, with the return shot directed down the alley. Being able to pass an opponent at the net down the alley is demoralizing, as that is the one area the net player must protect.

Angled cross-court returns and cross-court returns at the onrushing server's feet are exceptional choices for hitting winning shots. The server cannot reach angled cross-court shots unless the server anticipates the shot or the angled return lacks crispness. Cross-court shots at the feet of the server moving to the net catch the server in a tentative position, and the final result is often a ball hit up for an easy return volley.

The choice of which return to hit is controlled to a large extent by placement of the serve in the service court, and by the velocity of the serve. A serve hit to the inside corner of the deuce service court usually eliminates the passing shot because of the central location of the ball. All other service returns from that location remain possible.

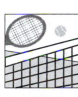

Doubles Game Plan and Strategy

The doubles plan of strategy is to (a) execute strokes in an attacking manner and (b) work to gain control of the net. All players at all levels of skill must do these two things. One of the easier skills in tennis is the volley shot. If a beginner can get to the net, play will be highly enjoyable from that position.

Once the concept of taking control of the net is ingrained, the doubles team must remember to protect the alley and middle of the court. The two must learn to move as a team, in tandem, supporting each other and retreating or advancing together. The receiving team must return serves on a low trajectory with pace and attempt to hit a predetermined target area. The serving team should establish a relentless plan of attack with the server coming to the net following a wellpaced serve.

Doubles play also requires specific responsibilities of each player during the serve. The server has the responsibility to get the first serve in play consistently to establish a flow, and to put pressure on the receiving team to return service effectively. The receiver of a serve in doubles must get the ball back across the net in play.

Once a beginner has developed the confidence to hit the ball back as receiver of a serve, it helps to think through a tactic or placement of the ball in advance, and to be ready for any type of serve. Net players on both the serving and receiving teams have similar responsibilities. Both have to be active and willing to poach. The players at the net also must have the courage to stand up and face a return of a shot and go on the attack rather than respond passively.

A final strategy is to communicate with the partner, out-think the opposing team, and out-reach the opponent. Communication is of particular importance. Teammates in doubles have to move in sync with each other. They need to verbally, or through hand signals, indicate what they are going to do. Today, more often than not, advanced players communicate verbally what type of serve they are going to hit and to what part of a service court. The net player conveys strategy at the net, including a preconceived plan to poach. Beginning players are not ready to be this sophistocated in their communication, but simple verbal responses on what to do next can aid doubles strategy.

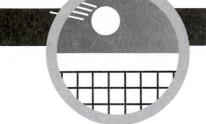

Points to Remember

Doubles Strategy

1. A two-back doubles formation is a defensive alignment that positions players behind the baseline when net skill is weak or the opponents are at the net hitting overheads.

2. Although a one-up, one-back formation is often used, it is highly vulnerable to open-area winning shots.

3. A two-up doubles tandem provides the most effective offensive alignment in doubles.

4. The Australian formation and I-formation provide a different alignment for the opposing team.

5. Getting your first serve in is critical in doubles.

6. Return of service requires hitting at the feet of the net player or the in-rushing server, passing the net player, lobbing the net players, or hitting cross-court angled toward the server.

7. The key to successful doubles is gaining control of the net.

Checkpoints ✔✔

1. With the exception of one choice, the two-back doubles formation is used
   a. as an offensive strategy by experienced players.
   b. as a defensive strategy by experienced players.
   c. as a beginning player alignment in doubles.
   d. by unskilled net players.

2. With the exception of one choice, the one-up, one-back doubles formation is used by
   a. experienced players.
   b. social players.
   c. novice players.
   d. mixed-doubles players.

3. A poach shot is a movement pattern in doubles defined as
   a. attempting to hit a winning volley shot.
   b. hitting a winning overhead.
   c. hitting a winning volley shot.
   d. attempting to hit a winning overhead.

4. Tandem play in doubles requires that
   a players move to the net together in an attacking mode.
   b. players move to the baseline in a defensive effort to retrieve a lob.
   c. players cover for each other but remain balanced on the court.
   d. all three strategies are accurate.

5. The strength of using an Australian doubles formation is to
   a. protect the baseline.
   b. protect against the lob.
   c. eliminate a cross-court return by the opponents.
   d. eliminate a down-the-line return.

6. Return of serve requires the receiver in doubles to
   a. hit at the feet of the server.
   b. pass the net player.
   c. lob the net player.
   d. do none of the above.

7. A two-back doubles formation is
   a. an offensive alignment.
   b. a containing alignment.
   c. a defensive alignment.
   d. all of the above.

8. When a doubles team is at the net, the reaction to a lob is to
   a. retreat straight back to return lob.
   b. designate one player who will retreat back and return lob.
   c. initiate a cross-action movement with the partner who can see the ball retreating to hit the return, and his teammate to cross over to the other side.
   d. any of the three are acceptable.

Answers to Checkpoints can be found on page 147.

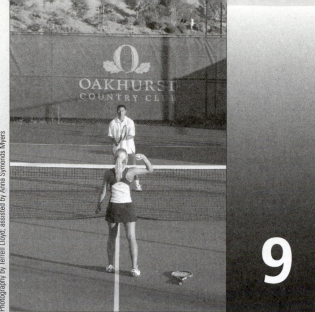

Photography by Terrell Lloyd; assisted by Anna Symonds Myers

9

Tennis Practice

Practice in between playing matches is good for developing tennis skills and applying them. Any group-instruction class uses numerous drills to develop skill. Reinforcement comes from playing in class and from suggestions during the performance of each drill-and-play situation. The beginning tennis player needs more work than can be provided in a group-instruction situation, however, and that work or practice can be achieved in additional practice time.

Development of muscle memory by hitting lots of balls correctly is critical to skill development. In one type of practice, you can do a series of drills by yourself; you don't need a partner. A second series of drills is designed for use with a partner so you can engage in rally and skill development situations that provide opportunities to test your skills and learn from your mistakes.

Tennis by Yourself

Tennis by yourself involves drills that require no partner, develops strokes with checkpoint of mechanics reminders, and encourages variation in drill selection. On many occasions a player cannot find a suitable partner or one who wants to practice. The drills presented, when done in detail, will take 45 minutes. They will give you a good physical workout and provide you with a skill practice session that you can do on your own. These individual drills are designed for progression. The more skills that are learned, the more drills that can be incorporated into practice.

Serving Drill

In the *serving* practice drill, the player uses 30 tennis balls and

CHECKPOINT OF MECHANICS
Serving Drill

Counting successful serves might be insightful, but total concentration on mechanics will be more productive.

1. Am I looking at the tennis ball on the toss?
2. Is my toss accurate? High enough? In line?
3. Are my feet where they belong?
4. Do I have a full backswing? Follow-through?
5. Is my grip appropriate to my serve?
6. Am I accurate? Why?

CHECKPOINT OF MECHANICS
Groundstroke Drill

1. Am I looking the ball into the racket?
2. Am I transferring weight into the ball?
3. Do I have a full backswing? Follow-through?
4. Am I hitting with the appropriate grip?
5. Am I turning my shoulder early?
6. Is the ball at least 5 feet high on the wall board?
7. Am I accurate? Why?

CHECKPOINT OF MECHANICS
Approach Shot Drill

1. Am I letting the ball drop, and am I timing my strokes?
2. Am I looking the ball into my racket?
3. Am I transferring my weight?
4. Is my backswing shortened?
5. Am I hitting into the court? Why?

serves to targets. The level of skill will establish the type of serves hit, and through a series of six sets, the player will hit 180 tennis serves.

Set #1   Serve 30 balls to the **ad service court**—inside corner.

Set #2   Serve 30 balls to the **deuce service court**—inside corner.

Set #3   Serve 30 balls to the ad service court—outside corner.

Set #4   Serve 30 balls to the deuce service court—outside corner.

Set #5   Serve 30 balls to the ad service court—10 to the outside, 10 to the middle, 10 to the inside.

Set #6   Serve 30 balls to the deuce service court—10 to the outside, 10 to the middle, 10 to the inside.

Movement Requirement   The player must run to the other side of the court and retrieve balls in a pickup run fashion.

Variations   Variations are quite acceptable, but only one type of serve per set should be initiated. A good variation is to serve and to go to the net for a volley, stopping as the ball strikes the service court.

Groundstroke Drill

The second drill—a simple **groundstroke**—uses a wall board, but goals must be set through the sequence. The drill has nine sets, each lasting 60 seconds. After each stroke the player must return to ready position and allow a distance to permit the ball to bounce twice before each stroke.

Set #1   Hit repetitive forehands.

Set #2   Hit repetitive backhands (remember to self-drop on the backhand side).

Set #3   Alternate forehand and backhand.

Sets #4, 5, and 6   Repeat sets 1–3 with slice.

Sets #7, 8, and 9   Repeat sets 1–3 with topspin.

Approach Shot Drill

Although designed for a more advanced tennis shot for a beginner, the third drill focuses on developing confidence and eliminating over-anxiety in players hitting *approach shots*. In practice, approach shots seldom are executed, so hitting four sets of 30 balls each will provide a good mental inset. Aim at the **service court line** for depth and 4 foot in from the sideline for accuracy (Figure 9.1). Drop the balls at least 2 feet away and at least waist high.

Set #1   From middle of the right service court, hit forehand down the line.

Set #2   From middle of the left service court, hit backhand down the line.

Set #3   From middle of the right service court, hit forehand cross-court.

Set #4   From middle of the left service court, hit backhand cross-court.

Movement Requirement   Player must run to the other side of the court and retrieve balls in a pickup run fashion.

Variations   The type of shot can be varied. The basic groundstroke pattern can be used, but as topspin and slice strokes are developed, they should be incorporated into the drill. Hitting topspin **down the line** is another variation of the drill. Also, placing the ball on the drop in different areas of the service court and between the baseline and the service court line contributes to variation.

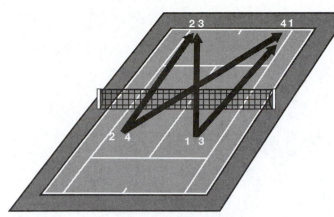

Figure 9.1 Approach shot movement drill.

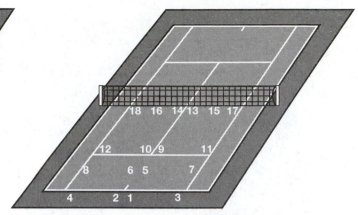

Figure 9.2 Shadow boxing movement, Set #1.

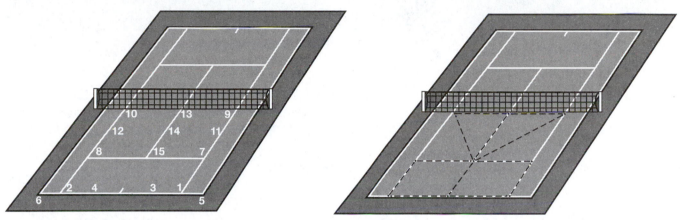

Figure 9.3 Shadow boxing movement, Set #2.

Figure 9.4 Fitness movement drill, Set #3.

CHECKPOINT OF MECHANICS

Overhead Drill

1. Am I timing my stroke in a smooth, rhythmical motion?
2. Is my backswing in the middle of my shoulder blades and my elbow up at a right angle?
3. Is my non-racket hand pointing in reference to the ball?
4. Am I hitting into the court? Why?

Moving Drill

A tennis player must *move*. Coupled with agility and quickness, movement can aid the player in getting to the ball in time. Three sets are designed to encourage agility and quickness and use of the racket in shadow boxing.

Set #1 Move to imaginary numbers and, in sequence, shadow box a groundstroke, an approach shot, or a volley (Figure 9.2). All balls stroked up to the service line require the players to return to ready position on the baseline, and all balls between the service line and the net require the player to assume a ready position at the net in the middle.

Set #2 The same drill as above except the shadow boxing should consist of lobs from the baseline and overhead smashes from the net (Figure 9.3). Player must assume ready position on each stroke.

Set #3 Eliminate shadow boxing, and move along the lines of the court, touching each junction between two lines (Figure 9.4).

Overhead Drill

The final drill is an *overhead.* The exercise requires a simple bounce of the ball off the court and above the head, providing time for the player to get set underneath the ball and hit an overhead.

Set #1 Hit 15 overheads from the right middle service court.

Set #2 Hit 15 overheads from the left middle service court.

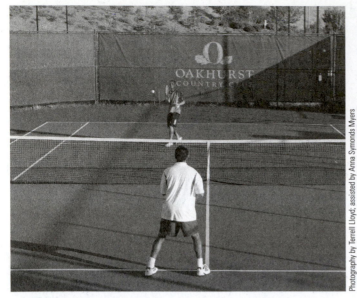

Photo 9.1 Short-court drill.

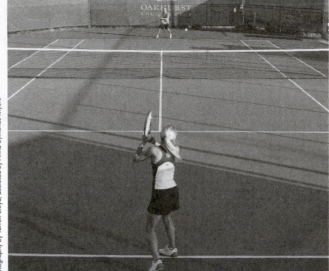

Photo 9.2 Bounce/hit drill.

Set #3 Hit 15 overheads from the right center position halfway between baseline and service line.

Set #4 Hit 15 overheads from the left center position halfway between baseline and service line.

Movement Requirement After each pair of sets, the player must run to the other side of the court and retrieve balls in a pickup run fashion.

Variations The player may locate other spots to hit the overhead and begin to identify the location of the target on the other side of the court.

The keys to executing the drills are to have a little self-discipline, become goal-oriented, and build confidence that each skill can be performed. Beginning players who participate three times per week in "tennis by yourself" will see a marked change in their skill development.

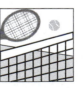

Partner Practice Drills

Partner practice drills supplement what you can practice on your own. Of the countless numbers of drills that involve two players, 14 are

presented in this chapter to provide a beginning approach to practice. Five of the drills are groundstroke-oriented because groundstrokes are the basis for the game. Additional drills will reinforce lobs, overheads, volley shots, and attacking the net.

Groundstroke Drills

Groundstroke drills progress from relatively simple drills designed to increase a beginner's skills.

Short-Court Drills The short-court drill is a "touch" drill that requires the partners to stand in the service court of their respective side and hit groundstrokes with touch (Photo 9.1). The idea is to keep the ball within the confines of the service court and to assist the player in anticipation, shoulder turn, and sensing the "feel" of the stroke.

Bounce/Hit Drill The bounce/hit drill (Photo 9.2) encourages focus and an inner feel for the groundstroke. The idea is for the partners to hit the ball from baseline to baseline without thinking about the mechanics of the stroke. By shouting "bounce" every time the ball bounces on the court and "hit" every time the ball is hit, the partners begin to focus on the ball and

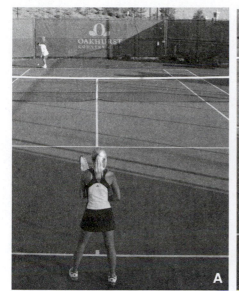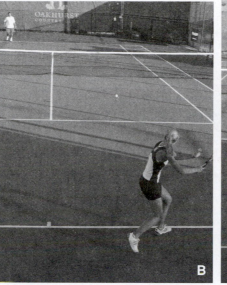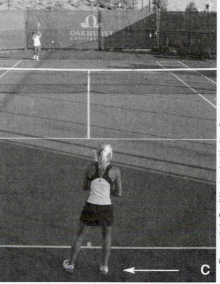

Photo 9.3 Homebase drill.

concentrate on the end result of hitting the ball to the other side of the court.

What is amazing is that form and mechanics of the groundstroke come about naturally when the partners become really involved in the drill. Two points to remember when executing this drill are:

1. Both partners must verbally identify "bounce" and "hit," regardless of which side of the net the ball is on.

2. The response must be loud enough for both partners to hear. Players tend to be self-conscious when doing this drill, and if there are players on adjacent courts, the etiquette of quiet on the courts might be disrupted. When used properly, however, this drill will truly be of help in skill development.

Homebase Drill The homebase drill requires the player to return to the baseline **center mark** after hitting each groundstroke. The underlying concept is that if the ball is hit deeply, it will keep the opposing player pinned to the baseline, restricting the player's ability to attack the net and thereby forcing errors (Photo 9.3A–C).

Both players are to use the area between the service court line and the baseline as the target for each shot hit. After hitting the groundstroke, that player must return to the baseline center mark area and prepare for the next groundstroke.

The drill is played under game-like situations in the sense that one player initiates play by self-dropping a groundstroke and hitting deep to the target area. A rally continues until one of the players hits a ball short of the target area. Play stops and the player who hits the short shot receives a negative point.

Play then resumes with another self-drop, followed by a groundstroke rally to the target area. Play continues to a set negative score, with the player accumulating the greater negative score declared the loser (the concept with deep rallies is that it is not so much a player winning a point but, rather, the other player losing the point).

As skill develops, challenges can be added to the drill. One example is to play a homebase-approach-shot game. When a ball is hit short of the depth target, the receiving player moves up to hit an approach shot. Hitting an approach force shot earns that player 1 point, but if the

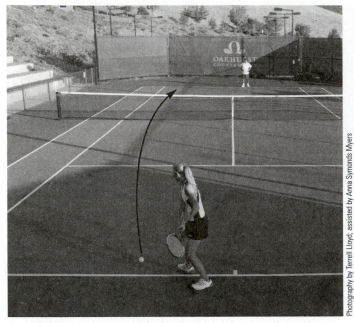

Photography by Terrell Lloyd; assisted by Anna Symonds Myers

Photo 9.4 Down-the-line groundstroke drill.

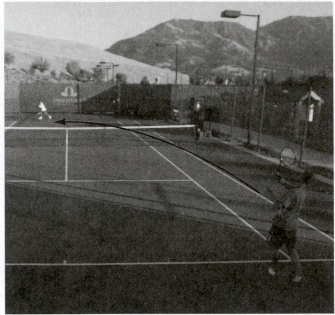

Photography by Terrell Lloyd; assisted by Anna Symonds Myers

Photo 9.5 Cross-court groundstroke drill.

shot is missed, a 2-point negative penalty is assigned to the player.

Increasing Beginner Skills: Down-the-Line Groundstroke Drill

Hitting down-the-line groundstrokes encourages the player to establish a target when hitting the ball (Photo 9.4). The idea is to hit the ball down the sideline to the partner. The ball should be positioned between the player and the sideline, forcing the player to hit a forehand or a backhand, depending on which is the appropriate shot (with two right-handed players, one would be hitting with a forehand, the other with a backhand groundstroke).

After hitting the ball, the player who has just hit returns to near the baseline center mark area. The idea is to have to move to hit the ball with the appropriate groundstroke rather than to stand in one spot, and eventually to play the ball so it is positioned for a choice of forehand or backhand.

Cross-Court Groundstroke Drill

The cross-court groundstroke drill has the same purpose of setting a target, and the same organizational setup, but instead of going down the line, the ball is hit cross-court

(Photo 9.5). Again, it is important to hit the ball and return to near the center mark.

These last two drills are somewhat difficult for beginners. They tend to become frustrated because they are uncomfortable with hitting a backhand and reaching the intended target. Increasing the level of this skill is important, however, and you will not improve if you don't push yourself.

Increasing Beginner Skills: Down-the-Line/Cross-Court Groundstroke Drill

The final groundstroke drill adds to the progression of difficulty because it combines *down-the-line with cross-court* (Photos 9.6A–D). The idea follows the sequence of:

1. Partner A hitting down the left sideline.

2. Partner B returning a cross-court shot to the right side court of Partner A.

3. Partner A then hitting down the right sideline to Partner B, who returns a shot cross-court to Partner A's left side court.

The sequence is repeated to develop consistency.

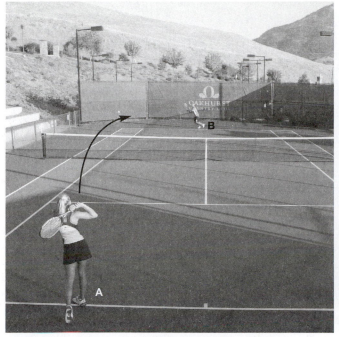

Photo 9.6A Down-the-line/cross-court drill sequence: Partner A hits down the left sideline.

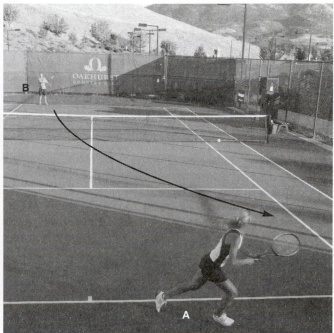

Photo 9.6B Down-the-line/cross-court drill sequence: Partner B returns a cross-court shot to the right side court of Partner A.

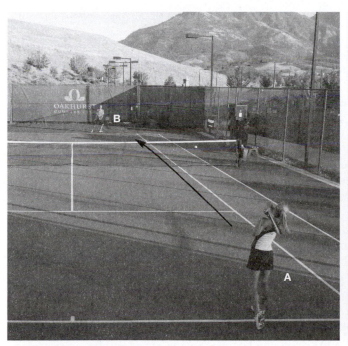

Photo 9.6C Down-the-line/cross-court drill sequence: Partner A hits down the right sideline to Partner B.

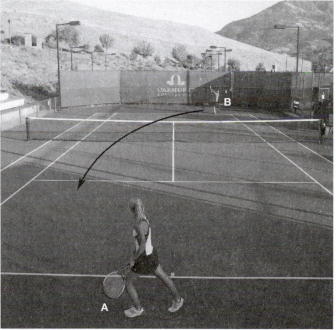

Photo 9.6D Down-the-line/cross-court drill sequence: Partner B returns a shot cross-court to Partner A's left side court.

Photography by Terrell Lloyd; assisted by Anna Symonds Myers

Lob/Overhead Drills

Lobs and overhead practice fit nicely together. Two drills—one incorporating a lob sequence, followed by a second, more advanced drill, consisting of a lob/overhead sequence—assists in developing these two skills.

Lob Sequence Drill   The *lob drill* simply requires the partners to exchange lobs (Photo 9.7). The

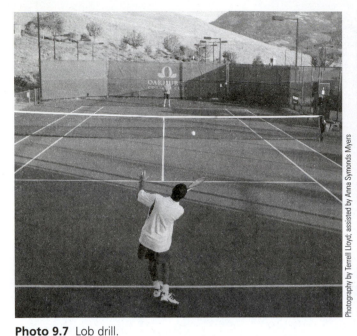

Photography by Terrell Lloyd; assisted by Anna Symonds Myers

Photo 9.7 Lob drill.

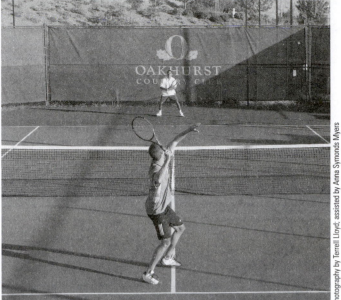

Photography by Terrell Lloyd; assisted by Anna Symonds Myers

Photo 9.8 Overhead sequence drill.

emphasis should be on hitting deep with proper height for the selected lob. You should start with a defensive lob and experiment with ball height, then continue by hitting topspin offensive lobs. Work on an equal number of forehand and backhand lobs, and as you progress, begin to place the lobs from corner to corner.

Increasing Beginner Skills: Lob/Overhead Sequence Drill

The second drill is an extension of the lob drill. It consists of an *overhead at the end of the lob* with one partner self-dropping and lobbing short to the service court area and the partner hitting overheads (Photo 9.8). As you improve, you should work on returning an overhead with a lob rather than self-dropping to initiate the partner's overhead shot.

Volley Drills

Two volley drills can enhance the skill of all players, including beginners: the *toss/volley* and the *face-to-face volley*. As skill develops two additional drills, designed to increase a beginner's skill, are included. They incorporate a *cross-step volley* and a *cross-court down-the-line volley*.

Toss/Volley Drill The toss/volley drill requires that one partner toss the ball to the other partner (Photo 9.9). The idea is to toss accurately to force the volleying partner to step into the ball with a short backswing and punch the ball back to the partner. This drill encourages good form, and it can progress with variations that force the volleying partner to hit low and high volleys as well as adjust to a ball at the body. In addition, the partner's toss can force the volleying partner to cross-step and punch the ball deep to the baseline.

Face-To-Face Volley Drill The face-to-face volley drill is a particularly fun drill because both partners face each other within their service courts and volley the ball back and forth (Photo 9.10). Progression again is important. Start with forehand-to-forehand volleys, then volley backhand to backhand. As your skill increases, you can alternate from forehand to backhand volleys, hit volleys at different elevations of the ball, and react to each placement of the ball that comes to you.

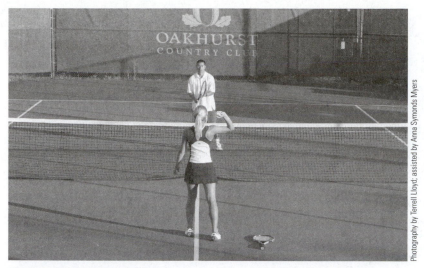

Photo 9.9 Toss/volley drill.

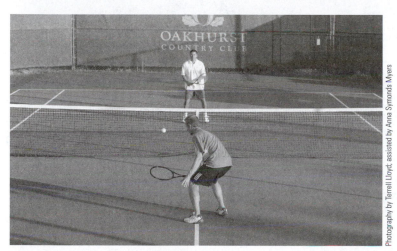

Photo 9.10 Face-to-face volley drill.

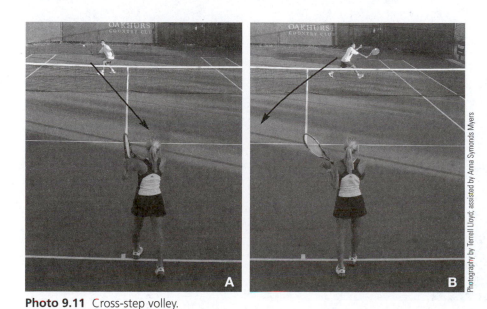

Photo 9.11 Cross-step volley.

Increasing Beginner Skills: Cross-Step Volley Drill The cross-step volley drill is designed to force the volleying player to cross-step rather than step with the inside foot (Photos 9.11A and B). The baseline player hits a selected number of groundstrokes wide to the forehand of the net player, and the net player cross-steps to hit a deep volley return. Then the baseline player hits the same number of groundstrokes to the backhand side, forcing cross-step volley returns. All volley returns are to be hit deep between the service court line and baseline.

Increasing Beginner Skills: Down-the-Line/Cross-Court Volley Drill The down-the-line/cross-court volley drill (Photos 9.12A–D) has the same premise as the cross-step volley drill illustrated in Photos 9.11A and B. The difference is that a select number of groundstrokes hit from the baseline are to be volleyed cross-court from the forehand side, then from the backhand side, and repeated with forehand down-the-line and backhand down-the-line shots.

Service Return Drill

Service returns seldom are practiced and, as a result, returns are neglected. The drill is simple: One partner serves and the other returns the serve (Photo 9.13). Focus on returns should be a first priority, with the main goal to hit each serve deep to the baseline. Then service returns can become more target-oriented by hitting both cross-court and down-the-line returns.

To become really skilled in return of service, the return partner should have the opportunity to return serves of different velocities with different spins. The drawback to practicing with another beginner is that neither is at the level to execute a variety of consistent serves. This drill requires a skilled partner to deliver the serves.

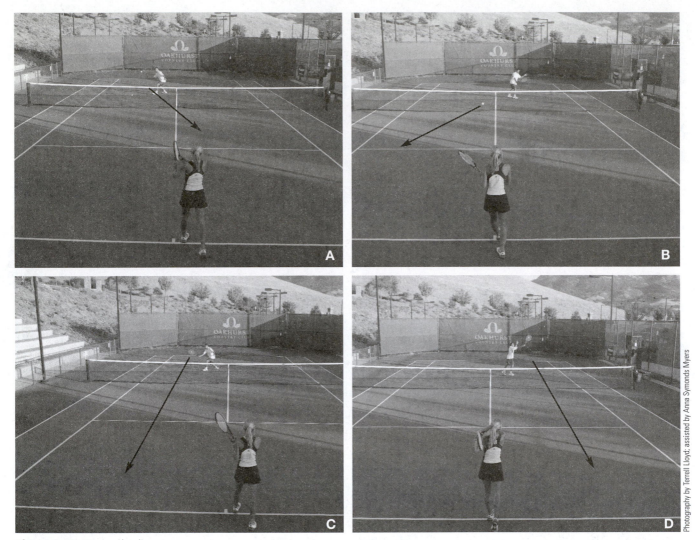

Photography by Terrell Lloyd; assisted by Anna Symonds Myers

Photo 9.12 Down-the-line cross court.

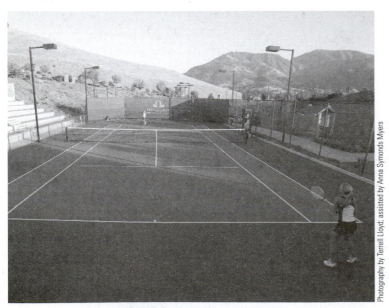

Photography by Terrell Lloyd; assisted by Anna Symonds Myers

Photo 9.13 Service return drill.

Increasing Beginner Skills: Attacking-the-Net Drill The final drill is an attacking-the-net drill designed for the beginner who is comfortable moving to the net. In this drill, one of the partners feeds the ball to the attacking partner. The feeding partner holds three balls and places the first ball deep to the forehand of the attacking partner. The attacking partner hits a deep forehand groundstroke return and begins to advance to the net. The feeding partner then places the second ball to the attacking partner's forehand, forcing a forehand approach shot deep to the baseline. The attacking partner continues to advance to the net and receives a

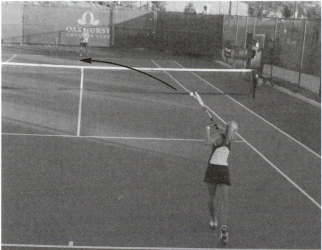

Photo 9.14A Attacking-the-net drill sequence: Attacking player hitting groundstroke.

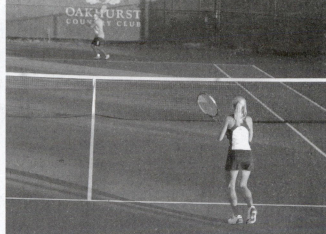

Photo 9.14B Attacking-the-net drill sequence: Attacking player moving forward.

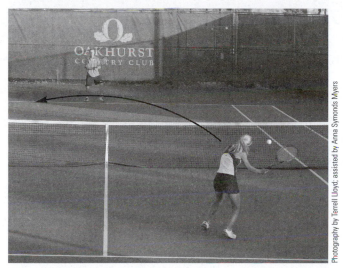

Photo 9.14C Attacking-the-net drill sequence: Attacking player returning volley shot.

Photography by Terrell Lloyd; assisted by Anna Symonds Myers

ball to the forehand side from the feeder that then is volleyed by the attacking partner (see Photos 9.14 A–C).

The sequence can be repeated to the backhand, and mixed so the attacking partner does not know which direction the ball is being placed. Other shots, including a second volley and an overhead, can be incorporated into the drill as skill improves. The attacking player also can work on placement with depth and at angles to gain the best advantage at the net. This is not a particularly easy drill, but you will be surprised how well you do because

you do not have time to think and because the ball is being placed to you.

The nice thing about tennis practice is that besides these 14 drills, there are even more options. The use of a ball machine allows for stroke consistency when it comes to hitting groundstrokes, volleys, lobs, and overheads. In Chapter 12, p. 138, the *International Book of Tennis Drills* is referenced for your use. It contains many good drills that will enhance your skill.

You can even design your own drills by using imagination and creativity. Practice is important. The practice-by-yourself and partner-practice drills will enable you to progress and increase your skill level more rapidly than by simply listening to instructions and practicing only during that instructional time. Once you gain the skills to play tennis, it is an easy game. Practice enables you to gain the skills so you can have fun.

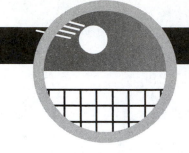

Points to Remember

Tennis Practice

1. It is critical to have meaningful practice following lessons and as a supplement to playing matches.

2. The "Tennis by Yourself" drills require effort and motivation to be helpful. To make the drills work, be sure you read the boxes related to each skill area.

3. Partner practice drills require a motivated partner who can return various shots with consistency.

Checkpoints ✔✔

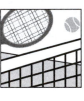

Select three specific skill related drills and describe how each drill will enhance your specific skill development.

_____

_____

_____

_____

_____

_____

_____

_____

_____

_____

_____

_____

_____

_____

_____

_____

Answers to Checkpoints can be found on page 147.

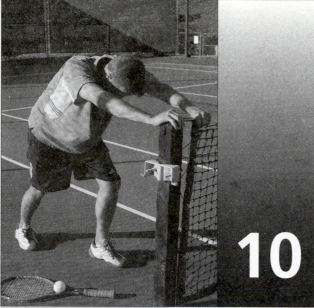

10

Physical Aspects of Playing Tennis

The physical aspects of playing tennis begin to take on a major role in performance when you can maintain a rally— keeping the ball in play for a significant amount of time. You need to be physically fit to play tennis. To do this, you should engage in an overall fitness-development program. As part of this program, you should be aware of how to prevent and care for tennis-related injuries and how to deal with problems on a tennis court related to heat, sun, and insects. And tennis playing should be preceded by a **warm-up** and followed by a **warm-down** period.

Warm-up

In preparation for play, the muscles should be engaged in some physical work. The work prescribed is an 8- to 10-minute warm-up, consisting of low-intensity jogging or cycling, which increases the blood flow, heart rate, and oxygen available to the muscles.

This low-intensity activity is followed by two phases of stretching: (1) stretching exercises as a warm-up to hitting the ball, and (2) the basic stroke warm-up. When stretching, young adult players tend to give a cursory effort to muscle readiness. But the body needs to establish a stretching routine that will be incorporated into the total playing habit into middle age and beyond.

The recommended *stretching exercises* include some **ballistic movement** along with **static stretching**. Devoting just 5 minutes to these warm-up efforts reduces the risk of injury, and relaxes the body in preparation for the competitive situation.

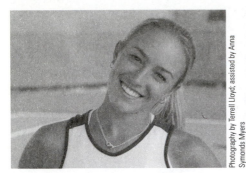

Photography by Terrell Lloyd; assisted by Anna Symonds Myers

Lateral Head Tilt

Action: Tilt the head slowly and gently to one side and hold the stretch for a few seconds. Alternate to the other side and repeat.

Areas Stretched: Flexors and extensors and ligaments of the cervical spine.

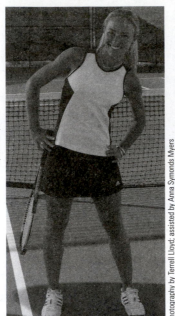

Photography by Terrell Lloyd; assisted by Anna Symonds Myers

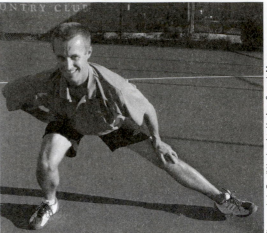

Photography by Terrell Lloyd; assisted by Anna Symonds Myers

Adductor Stretch

Action: Feet spread twice shoulder-width and hands placed slightly above the knee. Flex one knee and go down to approximately 90 degrees. Hold the stretch and then repeat on the other side.

Area Stretched: Hip adductor muscles.

Side Stretch

Action: Feet spread at shoulder width with hands on hips. Rotate the body to one side and repeat the process to the other side. Hold the stretch for a few seconds on each side.

Areas Stretched: Pelvis area muscles and ligaments.

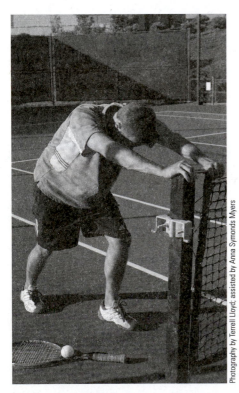

Photography by Terrell Lloyd; assisted by Anna Symonds Myers

Heel Cord Stretch

Action: Stand against a solid object and stretch the heel downward. Hold the stretch for a few seconds and change legs.

Areas Stretched: Achilles tendon, gastrocnemius and soleus muscles.

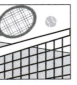

Stretching Exercises

Stretching exercises should begin with concentration on stretching neck flexors and extensors, ligaments of the cervical lumbar spine, ligaments of the shoulder joint, deltoid and pectoral muscles, abdominal muscles, muscles of the hip, muscles and ligaments of the pelvic area, quadriceps and hamstring of the upper leg, gastrocnemius and soleus muscles of the lower leg, and the Achilles tendon.

Eleven recommended stretching exercises for tennis are presented here. Each is described by the action required for execution and identified by the area to be stretched. Most of these exercises are extrapolated from Werner W. K. Hoeger's *Lifetime Physical Fitness & Wellness: A Personalized Program* (Thompson Learning, 2003.)

The range of the stretch is to be done within your comfort zone, and the intensity of the stretch never should be painful. Finally, the duration of a stretch should be for only a few seconds.

Basic Stroke Warm-up

The *basic stroke warm-up* follows the stretching exercises. This warm-up is designed to increase circulation and respiration, and to provide a grooving of tennis strokes. A good stroke warm-up should last a total of 15 minutes, and at the conclusion, both players should be perspiring. When warming up, the beginning player should always work on strokes

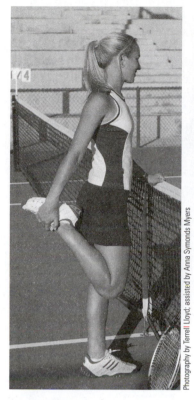

Photography by Terrell Lloyd; assisted by Anna Symonds Myers

Quad Stretch

Action: Stand up straight, grasp the front of the ankle and flex the knee until the heel of the foot is touching the gluteal area. Hold the stretch for a few seconds, then change legs.

Areas Stretched: Quadriceps muscle, and knee and ankle ligaments.

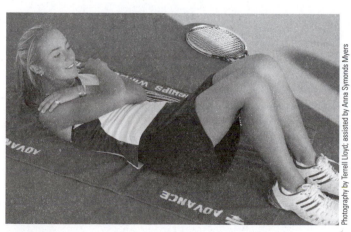

Photography by Terrell Lloyd; assisted by Anna Symonds Myers

Curls

Action: Lie flat on padded surface and bend knees at a 90-degree angle. Place the arms across chest and curl the upper body to the knees. Repeat the process 15–20 times.

Area Exercised: Abdominal muscles.

Photography by Terrell Lloyd; assisted by Anna Symonds Myers

Single-Knee to Chest Stretch

Action: Lie flat on a padded surface. Bend one leg at approximately 100 degrees and place both hands on the lower portion of the knee of the opposite leg, pulling that knee toward the chest. Hold the stretch at chest level.

Area Stretched: Lower back and hamstring muscles, and the lumbar spine ligaments.

Photography by Terrell Lloyd; assisted by Anna Symonds Myers

to be used in the match. The players should be partners in the warm-up—giving as well as receiving, and attempting to ensure that the other partner has had the opportunity for a sound warm-up. The sequence for every tennis warm-up is as follows:

1. Groundstrokes.

2. One player hits groundstrokes, the other volleys, then switch.

3. One player hits lobs while the other hits overheads, then switch.

4. One player hits serves while the other player retrieves the serves, then switch. (Note: there is no return of service; that takes time and detracts from the total warm-up effort.)

Although the sequence may differ depending on the location of the players and the player skill level, the concept is reasonably standard.

Warm-down

At the conclusion of the match and while the players are talking to each other, they should complete a *warm-down*. The warm-down stretching exercises identified include:

1. Side stretch.

2. Adductor stretch.

3. Heel cord stretch.

4. Quad stretch.

As part of the warm-down, assuming it is not extremely hot, put on a warm-up top and pants and cool down by stretching and walking for a period of time prior to sitting down for a rest. While stretching and walking, make sure to continue drinking liquids. If you have an injury or muscle soreness, apply an ice pack on that area for 15–20 minutes.

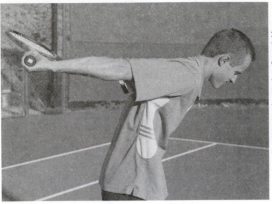

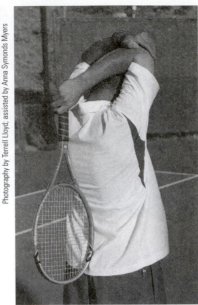

Photography by Terrell Lloyd; assisted by Anna Symonds Myers

Photography by Terrell Lloyd; assisted by Anna Symonds Myers

Shoulder Hyperextension Stretch

Action: Grasp the throat of the racket with hands close together. Slowly bring the arms up to as close to a perpendicular position to the shoulders as possible. Hold the stretch for a few seconds.

Areas Stretched: Deltoid and pectoral muscles and ligaments of the shoulder joint.

Serving Shoulder and Arm Stretch

Action: Place the tennis racket head in the small of the back with the elbow in an up position. Place the non-racket hand below the elbow and apply minimal pressure to place the shoulder area on stretch. Hold the stretch for a few seconds and repeat the process several times.

Areas Stretched: Ligaments of the shoulder joint and ligaments of the cervical and lumbar spine.

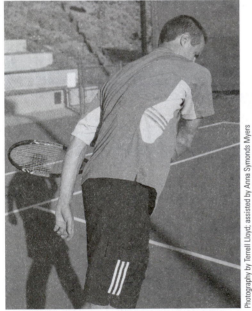

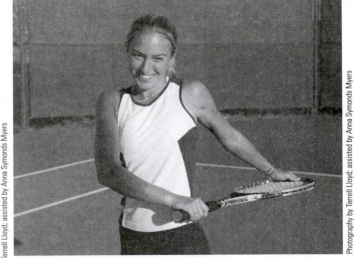

Photography by Terrell Lloyd; assisted by Anna Symonds Myers

Photography by Terrell Lloyd; assisted by Anna Symonds Myers

Serving Motion Rotation and Stretch

Action: Start with the head of the tennis racket between the shoulder blades, and rotate through the service motion. Hold the stretch on the follow-through for a few seconds and repeat the process.

Areas Stretched: Upper and lower back area.

Semi-Groundstroke Body Rotation

Action: Place the feet approximately shoulder-width apart, grasp the racket with your hands, and with the arms away from the body, rotate the trunk as far as possible and hold the stretch. Repeat the rotation the other direction, and continue to follow the same process several times.

Areas Stretched: Hips, abdominal, chest, back, neck, shoulder muscles, and hip spinal ligaments.

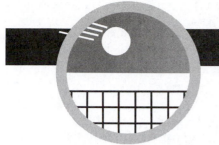

Points to Remember

Physically Preparing to Play

1. Do physical work for 8–10 minutes before stretching.
2. Stretching exercises should include both upper and lower body.
3. The tennis stroke warm-up consists of a sequence of groundstrokes, volleys, lobs/overheads, and service.
4. After a match, warm down by walking and stretching, while continually taking in liquids, and icing sore muscles.

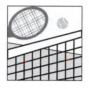

Developing Overall Fitness

Fitness development for tennis can range from basic to sophisticated through the use of aerobic exercise and strength training programs. Tennis players who are willing to run, follow a sensible exercise program, and work on tennis drills that incorporate agility and quickness will establish an advantage over individuals who neglect fitness development.

Developing Aerobic Fitness

Aerobic exercise contributes significantly to success as a tennis player. You cannot use your skills and apply strategy to your best advantage if you are not in good physical shape. In addition, you are at risk for potential injury. During a tennis rally most of the energy the body uses is a product of anaerobic metabolism, the release of energy without the use of oxygen.

Therefore, although energy needs during tennis play are not primarily **aerobic** ("with oxygen"), the more oxygen that can be used during a rally, the faster you can

recover and the less tired you will be during play. This means that you need to train your body to use large amounts of oxygen quickly. You can accomplish this through a number of physical activities, but a jogging program is recommended, as tennis is a running form of activity.

For most people under age 35, an exercise intensity between 70 percent and 85 percent of *maximal heart rate* is adequate and is called an *exercise heart rate range*. Maximal heart rate is the fastest a heart can beat when exercising as hard as you can. The typical way to predict your exercise heart rate range is to take the number 220 and subtract your age. After you have tabulated that number, simply multiply 70 percent and 85 percent of that number. For example:

$$220 - 20 \text{ years of age} = 200$$
$$200 \times 70\% = 140$$
$$200 \times 85\% = 170$$

Calculation of these two numbers represents an exercise heart rate range (i.e., a 20-year-old's exercise heart rate range is between 140 and 170). If you are in good health, this heart rate range will provide a guide for your level of exercise effort. Also, before starting any exercise program, it is advisable to have a physical exam.

Once you have arrived at a proper rate of exercise intensity, you have to determine the duration of your workout effort. Anywhere between 15 and 60 minutes will provide enough time to give your body sufficient practice at using oxygen. In general, 20–30 minutes is recommended as the proper workout duration. This means 20–30 minutes of constant, nonstop exercise at your exercise heart rate. If you are just starting out, you need to progressively work into a full workout. It does you no good to start at a high level of effort only to experience discomfort or injury the first day. Start slowly and progress to a more full workout. Try to do your aerobic work at least three or four times per week. Five times per week can be tolerated, but you also need to give your body a chance to rest. A minimum of 24 hours between aerobic workouts is desirable. The less fit you are, the more time you need to set aside between your aerobic work and rest.

If you combine aerobic work with practice time on the tennis court using the drills presented in Chapter 9, *Tennis Practice*, you will gain a positive level of fitness and also you will have improved your quickness and agility for tennis play.

Developing Strength and Fitness

Several forms of *strength training* are designed for further development of both muscular strength and endurance, which can also enhance physical development for tennis. You can use either free weights or weight machines to accomplish this development. Each of these workouts should include weight work for shoulder strength, abdominal development, bicep and tricep strength, quadricep and hamstring strength development, and calf strength development. When you do these exercises, you should breathe, and lift, using a smooth, slow action.

Your workouts should consist of a minimum of 3 days per week with 2–3 sets of 10–15 repetitions. One of the exciting aspects of strength-training programs is that most colleges and universities have established facilities for your choice of weight-training workout, with state-of-the-art equipment.

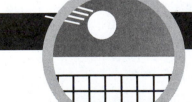

Points to Remember

Overall Fitness Development

1. Predict an exercise heart rate range by subtracting your age from 220, then multiplying that number by 70% and 85% to determine a range.

2. Aerobic workouts should consist of 20–30 minutes for 3 or 4 times per week.

3. Strength training workouts using weight-training machines should consist of 2–3 sets of 10–15 repetitions each.

Preventing and Caring for Tennis Injuries

Of the numerous injuries associated with tennis, most can be prevented. Serious injuries related to contact sports, including concussions, cartilage and ligament damage of the knee, shoulder separations, and neck injuries, are seldom found in tennis. Knee, shoulder, and back injuries, however, are increasing in number. Hard tennis court surfaces can be blamed for many knee and back injuries, and overuse or improper shoulder rotation when serving often contributes to shoulder injuries.

As a general rule, injuries in tennis usually are mild and seldom restrict a player's participation. The few serious injuries that do occur can be prevented in many cases.

Minor Tennis Injuries

Some common minor tennis injuries can be prevented with a little attention.

Blisters The blisters that often appear on the hands and feet are caused by moisture, pressure, or friction. Blisters on the feet are caused by the feet sliding in tennis shoes. To prevent these blisters, wear cotton tennis socks with cushion insoles.

Blisters on the racket hand often are caused by the racket turning in the player's hand. You can prevent this type of blister by making sure you have the correct grip size. Usually a larger grip enables a player to prevent the racket from turning in the hand. Blisters also develop on the racket hand from extensive play when the hand has not been accustomed to that amount of play. The wear and tear creates a "hot spot" that results in a blister. Prevention consists of being conscious of length of playing time and placing some limit on it.

Bruises Sometimes a player is bruised when hit by a ball or racket. The only way to avoid this injury is to avoid positions on the court that provide an opportunity to be hit, or to avoid being hit in vulnerable spots of the body. For example, if you are on the direct opposite side of the net from the opposing player and the opposing player is about to hit an overhead in line with your position on the court, it is prudent for you to turn and duck.

Also, bruising can occur when a player follows through with the racket and hits the shin when serving, or when doubles partners swing at the same ball and hit each other. These incidents can cause severe bruising, called a *hematoma*.

Cramps In unusually warm and humid weather, when a person loses body fluid and salt rapidly, a player may get cramps. A muscle or muscle group contracts, causing spasms, usually in the abdominal area or gastrocnemius (calf muscle). To prevent a serious cramping problem, consume fluids in large quantities. Although water is the best choice of liquids, diluted fruit juices are an excellent alternative. Sports drinks (such as Gatorade®, Powerade®, and Exceed®) also are alternatives to dealing with cramps, as they replace carbohydrates and electrolytes while also replenishing liquid. The key to liquid consumption on a hot, humid day is to drink, and then drink more ("Drink a Sports Drink?" *Tennis,* July 1996 p. 99).

More Serious Tennis Injuries

The following more serious tennis injuries require professional care.

Pulled Muscles Pulled muscles, including the groin, hamstring, and gastrocnemius, usually occur as a result of poor stretching preparation. These injuries often can be avoided by going through a full warm-up. You will know when you have pulled a muscle simply from the pain and limited mobility following the pull.

Common remedies are rest, ice, and other athletic training modalities. If you pull a muscle, it is important to see a sports-medicine-oriented physician or athletic trainer for evaluation.

Sprained Ankles A sprained ankle is one of the most common injuries in tennis. These injuries usually happen when the player tries to make a quick turn without the foot following in the turn. Sometimes a player jumps to hit a ball with a scissors kick on the overhead and lands on the side of the foot, or a player steps on a ball during play. Pivoting incorrectly or landing on the side of the foot is a matter of not coordinating effort and physical skill.

Stepping on the ball is controllable. Only three tennis balls should be available for play at any given point in a match. If one ball is in play during a rally, only two other balls can become a problem. Court awareness is important. You should keep your side of the court "clean" by picking up or pushing balls on the court to the net or fence. You also should be aware of a ball that comes from another court and stop play if the ball is in your court area. If a tennis player is lazy when it comes to picking up loose tennis balls, injury can be the result.

Ankle sprains are classified as Grade 1 (painful), Grade 2 (very painful), and Grade 3 (severe pain). Most ankle sprains occur to the outside of the ankle. With any significant discomfort, the player should see a physician for an x-ray, and once identified as a sprain, you should begin using ice in combination with rest, elevation, and compression ("Twist and Shout," by A.

Shaffer, *Tennis*, June 1999, pp. 93–96). You don't recover from an ankle sprain overnight. Give yourself time to rehabilitate.

Foot Injuries Foot injuries occur in three of four people. If you play long enough, you will sustain a foot injury. *Plantar fasciitis* is a high-risk foot injury. Symptoms are pain in the heel or arch, usually after you have rested following playing.

Other foot injuries include inflammation of the sesamoid bone (the two metacarpal bones behind the big toe), capsulitis (an inflammation of connective tissue under the second toe), metatarsalgia (inflammation under the ball of the foot), tendonitis, stress fracture, and the common foot callus ("Foot Faults," by A.L. Shaffer, *Tennis*, May 2000, pp. 80–82).

Knee Injuries Tennis players are susceptible to knee injuries because of the weak anatomical structure of the knee and the quick lateral movements and countless stops and starts required during play. Typically, knee injuries are related to overuse and don't require surgery. Patellar tendonitis and patellofemoral pain syndrome are reflective of overuse and are treated with ice, rest, compression, and elevation. This combination speeds the healing process and reduces any tissue damage.

Shoulder Injuries The second most likely tennis injury consists of shoulder injuries. The shoulder relies on muscles, tendons, and ligaments to maintain stability, and tennis injuries tend to effect these soft tissues rather than the bones. Overuse injuries often occur in tennis with a player repetitively hitting with a serving motion or overhead. This causes a pinching of the rotator cuff tendons, which can result in tendonitis or bursitis, or more serious structural damage.

Symptoms suggesting a shoulder injury include pain and weakness in the shoulder (tendonitis), gradual onset of pain in the front and upper shoulder (bursitis), feeling that the arm has slipped out of its socket (dislocation), and the inability to raise the arm (torn rotator cuff). Each injury is treated differently. Tendonitis and bursitis require rest and ice application along with anti-inflammatory medication. A dislocation or torn rotator cuff requires medical intervention ("The Unknown Shoulder," *Tennis*, June 2001, pp. 65–68).

Wrist Injuries Wrist injuries are increasing in tennis. The most common are tendonitis of the extensor tendons of the back of the hand, trauma to the soft tissue triangular fibrocartilage that encircles the wrist, and a carpal ligament sprain. These injuries happen when the player is using a racket with limited shock absorption or too high string tension. Other causes are applying too much pressure with spin strokes (i.e., slice or topspin) or swinging late.

Wrist injuries can be managed through some modifications.

1. Either lower the tension on your racket strings or get a more flexible racket for better shock absorption.

2. If you are experiencing discomfort hitting spin shots, back off and return to basic strokes.

3. Work on stroke timing to make solid, timed contact with the ball.

Wrist injuries "grow" on you. When you first feel pain, it is time to stop and check it out. If you let pain continue, your wrist problems will expand. Rest and ice application are advised with a wrist injury. After 10 days without improving, it is time for you to go to a doctor. If you must play with a wrist injury, wrist braces are available, but you should make sure you are not developing a chronic injury before you go to a wrist brace.

Shin Splints The constant pounding, running, jumping, and landing on a hard court can create an inflammation of the soft tissues of the lower legs called shin splints. A change of tennis court surfaces, a high foot arch, tight calves, and intensity in your workouts and playing situations all can contribute to this injury. This injury is identified by pain along the front and sides of the shins.

Prevention requires being aware of the causes, stretching, and using common sense regarding playing intensity and type of court you are playing on. Selecting the proper shoe with arch support and excellent shock absorption capabilities is also important. Recommended ways of dealing with a shin splint injury are rest and the application of ice when shin splints are in the acute stage ("How to Prevent Shin Splints," by D. Higdon, *Tennis*, June 1992, p. 102).

Back Injury Tennis requires repetitive twisting and trunk rotation. The trunk accelerating through on groundstrokes and executing the overhead arching motion in a serve or overhead increase the risk for back injury. In addition, hard court surfaces can be damaging.

Preventive measures for back injury include aerobic conditioning, strength programs, and good stroke technique. Also, improving lower back and hamstring flexibility can save you from nagging back injuries. Professional help following a back injury includes rehabilitation provided by an athletic trainer or a physical therapist who specializes in sports medicine ("Oh, My Aching Back," by D. Squires, *Tennis USTA*, April 1993, p. 10).

Achilles Tendon Injuries The Achilles tendon sometimes is injured by simple physical actions such as jumping and landing on the ball of the foot without lowering the heel, or by pushing off the ball of the foot, thereby placing extreme pressure on the tendon. When rupturing, the tendon sounds like a gunshot, and the player becomes immobile immediately. Ridged, high-arched feet with heels that angle inward or flat feet that roll inward are most vulnerable to Achilles tendon problems.

The Achilles tendon often is chronically sore because players ignore persistent, tolerable pain and swelling and continue to play. The Achilles tendon and the sheath that surrounds it become inflamed, and soreness, swelling and pain are the outcome. Ignoring these signs can lead to severe problems. The only way to address the injury is to stop playing and rest. To prevent Achilles tendon injuries in the first place, the Achilles tendon should be stretched in warm-up and warm-down.

Orthotics for the shoe, or heel pads, also are used as a preventive measure, but elevating your heel also shortens the tendon when what is needed is to lengthen the tendon. As a result, stretching becomes even more important when using a heel pad.

Once an Achilles tendon injury has occurred, rehabilitation consists of rest and modality application. Possible modalities used in therapy include ice, massage, ultrasound, and electrical stimulation. They are used to reduce swelling and begin rehabilitation that brings the Achilles tendon back to a normal condition.

A stiff or achy tendon is a sign of an impending rupture. If you rupture an Achilles tendon, the process of rehabilitation following surgery or immobilization is lengthy ("Protecting Your Achilles," by A. McNab, *Tennis,* June 1993, p. 99).

Tennis Elbow Of the several types of tennis elbow injuries, the main characteristic is inflammation of the elbow area, usually recognized as nagging pain on the outside of the elbow or forearm. The injury can be prevented by using proper skill techniques and strokes and selecting a racket with proper tension, weight and grip size. Hitting with the elbow leading on the backhand or hitting numerous slice or spin serves especially invites the injury. Treatment of an elbow injury is restricted to rest or application of a support. Elbow supports and splints, along with icing the painful area 15–30 minutes, several times a day, and taking an anti-inflammatory medication such as ibuprofen are available to relieve minor pain from tennis elbow, but they will not eliminate the cause.

Treatment Resources

If an injury is perceived as serious, a physician should be consulted as soon as possible. Then, if rehabilitation is recommended, it is advisable to seek out a sports medicine clinic. Most metropolitan areas have centers that work closely with physicians to rehabilitate injuries.

Home treatment should be limited to only minor injuries. Blisters usually dry up on their own; the main concern is to make sure that they do not get infected. For minor injuries, athletic trainers can create devices to enable continuation of activity. For example, a trainer can devise a doughnut-shaped pad that will cover the blister, reduce pain at the pressure point, and prevent additional friction on the blister area. Bruises often can be treated with cold compresses or ice packs to reduce swelling. For injuries such as Achilles tendon, tennis elbow, and pulled muscles, rest may be the only solution.

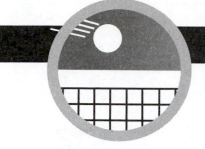

Points to Remember

Preventing and Caring for Tennis Injuries

1. Minor common tennis injuries include blisters, bruises, and cramps.
2. Serious tennis injuries include pulled muscles, sprained ankles, foot injuries, knee injuries, shoulder injuries, wrist injuries, shin splints, back injuries, Achilles tendon injuries, and tennis elbow.

Dealing with Heat, Sun, and Insect Bites, when Playing Tennis

Additional problems that arise in tennis include hyperthermia, dehydration, sunburn, and insect bites or stings.

Heat- and Sun-related Problems

Hyperthermia Hyperthermia (elevated body temperature) may lead to heat cramps, heat exhaustion, and heat stroke. Any of these conditions can occur when playing in hot weather for an extended time, because large amounts of body fluids are lost through sweating. *Heat cramps* can be painful, but they are not life-threatening. Untreated *heat stroke*, however, can be fatal.

Dehydration To prevent problems associated with *dehydration,* make sure your clothing allows for good air circulation around your body. Avoid clothing that traps or absorbs heat. Dark shirts are an example of material that absorbs heat. Wearing light clothing reduces that absorption.

Maintaining intake of body fluids is important in regulating body temperature. If too many fluids are lost,

the body is likely to overheat just like a radiator does when its water level is low. Some sweating is necessary to keep the body cool, so you need to replace lost fluids by drinking appropriate liquids. To determine how much liquid to drink, a good guide is to drink a pint of water for each pound lost during play. Start replacing your body fluids by drinking small (3–6 ounces of water) amounts in 10–15 minute intervals prior to beginning a match and continuing throughout the match. Because water is being lost from the body, water is needed to replace body fluids. Most people do not need electrolyte replacement solutions (such as Gatorade®) during exercise, although these fluids aid in recovery after play. You should avoid beverages with caffeine, as they contribute to dehydration.

Sunburn *Sunburn* can be avoided by applying sunscreen with a sun protection factor (SPF) of at least 15. PABA sunscreen offers even better protection. This type of sunscreen blocks both UVA and UVB rays. Wearing a hat is a prerequisite for avoiding sunburn and also for preventing heat stroke. Players often reject sunscreen because the lotion is applied by hand and then is transferred to the racket grip. By simply wiping your hands, you can avoid transferring the lotion to the grip of the racket. Some players also reject wearing a hat, suggesting that they can't see the ball on the serve toss and it gets in their way generally. These are just excuses.

Eye Conditions   One last potential physical problem deserves consideration. Eyes exposed to ultraviolet rays over an extended time are at risk for at least three eye diseases:

1. Cataracts (clouding of the lens),

2. Pterygium (a flesh-like growth on the white of the eye near the iris),

3. Macular degeneration (breakdown of the retina with age).

Pterygium is of particular concern, as the incidence of developing this eye disease is relatively high for those who are in the sun extensively ("The Eyes Have It," by K. Chen, *Tennis*, May 1995, p. 74). A partial answer is to begin wearing sunglasses while playing tennis. New technology has produced a polycarbonate lens, in which the lens is wrapped around the head. It is recommended that the lens block 100 percent of UVA rays and 75–90 percent of visible light ("Here Comes the Sun," by D. Sullivan, *Tennis*, July/August 1999, pp. 113–115). A quality pair of sunglasses protects against the sun and also screens out peripheral light and wind while still providing clear visibility for the player.

Insect Bites and Stings

Depending on what part of the country you come from, insect bites and stings might bother you. Probably the most prevalent insect sting is from bees or wasps. When you are around bees and wasps, be especially alert. When you pick up a racket, make sure a bee is not lurking. Bees and wasps congregate at the opening of cans containing beverages with sugar.

If you are stung, the recommended way of removing the stinger is to scrape the sac away and extract the stinger with a tweezer. Application of ice to the site also may be required to reduce swelling. If you are allergic to stings, you may have to seek immediate medical attention.

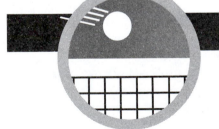

Points to Remember

Dealing with Heat, Sun, and Insects, when Playing Tennis

1. Drink water prior to playing and throughout a match.

2. Protect yourself from the sun by applying at least a 15 SPF sunblock.

3. Protect your eyes from the sun by wearing sunglasses with a lens block of 100 percent UVA and a 75–90 percent block of visible light.

4. Be alert to insects that sting—bees, wasps, etc.

Checkpoints ✔✔

1. Warm-up requires
   a. an increase in blood flow.
   b. an increase in heart rate.
   c. a series of stretching activities.
   d. all of the above.

2. Select a stretch action for the upper extremity and name the areas or muscles stretched:

   _____

   _____

   _____

3. Select a stretch action for the lower extremity and name the areas or muscles stretched:

   _____

   _____

   _____

4. Numerous possible injuries are associated with tennis. Three serious conditions are
   a. dehydration, tennis elbow, and back injuries.
   b. blisters, bruises, and dehydration.
   c. sprained ankles, shin splints, and Achilles tendon rupture.
   d. blisters, sprained ankles, and cartilage damage.

5. Determine your exercise heart rate by
   a. taking the number 220 and dividing by 70% and 85%.
   b. taking the number 220, dividing by your age and multiplying by 70% and 85%.
   c. taking the number 220, subtracting your age, and multiplying 70% and 85%.
   d. taking the number 220 and subtracting by 70 and 85.

6. Drinking liquids is important
   a. prior to and following a match.
   b. prior to, during, and following a match.
   c. prior to and during a match.
   d. during and following a match.

7. Tennis players usually are susceptible to knee injuries because of
   a. quick lateral movements and weak anatomical structure of the knee.
   b. sprinting and weak anatomical structure of the knee.
   c. jumping and weak anatomical structure of the knee.
   d. quick lateral movements and sprinting.

8. Sunglasses should be designed to
   a. block out 15 percent of UVA.
   b. block out 75 percent of UVA.
   c. block out all UVA.
   d. decrease as much as possible UVA.

Answers to Checkpoints can be found on page 147.

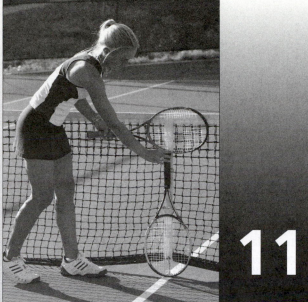

11

Tennis Behavior and Interpretation of Rules

The game of tennis has written and unwritten rules that the player must understand to play the game. Tennis has been played for centuries, and certain ways of behaving and interpreting rules have evolved over time.

Behavior on a Tennis Court

The unwritten rules of tennis prescribe behavior on a tennis court. Most have a logical reason or purpose, and it is up to the player to respect these rules.

Clothing

Appropriate clothing for tennis does not require a major expenditure, and proper dress is part of the game. A tennis player must wear tennis shoes rather than track-type shoes or basketball shoes. Wearing proper shoes reduces the chance of injury and also prevents marring of the tennis court surface (Chapter 12 contains additional comments about shoes as equipment). Municipal, private,

and college courts have basic, general rules requiring proper footwear, and, in addition, players are expected to wear shorts and a shirt to play on those courts. When playing at a private tennis club, clothing expectations are more conventional, consisting of tennis shorts or skirt and a tennis shirt or blouse.

Even the act of picking up a tennis ball requires a certain behavior. Bending over and picking up the ball is, of course, one way to retrieve the ball. Other methods include a foot/racket pickup and a ball-bounce pickup.

In the *foot/racket pickup* (Photo 11.1), the ball is positioned between the racket-side foot and the face of the tennis racket. Simultaneously lift the foot, ball, and racket to mid-calf level, and, as the ball becomes airborne, use the racket to bounce the ball to the court surface and catch it with your non-racket hand.

The *ball-bounce pickup* (Photo 11.2) requires you to choke up on the racket handle and place the racket face on top of the ball. Then lift the racket slightly and contact

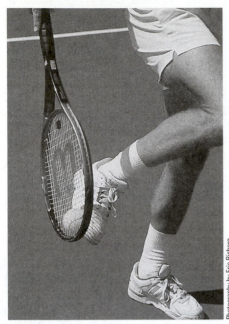

Photo 11.1 Foot/racket pickup.

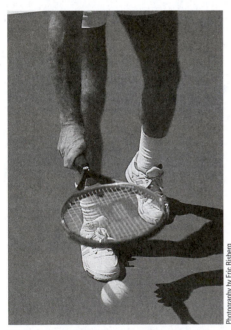

Photo 11.2 Ball-bounce pickup.

the ball with a series of quick wrist movements that lift the ball off the court and into your non-racket hand.

Walking and Talking on the Court

Most tennis facilities consist of three or more courts enclosed by a fence, with one or two gates to admit players. When walking on a tennis court, you should wait until any play has stopped before proceeding to an assigned court, and you should walk along the fence as quickly as possible.

Talking on a tennis court should be in normal voice tones. Conversation should be limited as much as possible to the match rather than to everyday visiting.

Warm-up

Warm-up is described in Chapter 10 as a part of physically preparing to play. Etiquette, or proper behavior, insists that each player be considerate during warm-up.

Return of Tennis Balls

How are you to return tennis balls to another court, and request a return of tennis balls? When a tennis ball rolls across a court from an adjacent court while play is in progress, action should stop and the ball should be returned. The action should be stopped, assuming that the rolling ball interferes with the play, and the point replayed. The ball should be returned to the adjacent court on a bounce to the requesting player.

If a ball is hit onto another court, the requesting player should wait until play ceases on that court, and then with a raised hand request "ball please," followed by "thank you" upon receiving the ball. Balls hit over the fence must be retrieved, and the retrieval should follow the same court behavior as when entering the court for the first time.

Ball in Play

Once the ball is in play during a match, interruptions should cease. This includes practice serves which are done as part of the warm-up. If practice serves are done during the first or second games of the match, they interfere with the flow of the game.

The server always must begin with two tennis balls. For convenience, one ball should be placed in the pocket of the tennis shorts and one in the hand for the toss. When receiving, the player should hit only a ball that is legally in play. Returning an "out" serve is poor form.

When a ball or other interference occurs during a match, a gesture of "play a let" is acceptable. In one situation the server hits the first serve as fault, followed by a ball rolling across the court. If the receiver responds by picking up the ball and returning it to the adjacent court, the receiver should immediately respond to the server, "Take two."

Another form of court behavior is to communicate all calls to the opponents. Verbal forms of communication are "out" and "let." A ball that is "in" is assumed in by the continued play on the part of the player who is returning the shot. An index finger pointing up can be used as sign language indicating that a ball is out, and a ball hit out of reach of a player that is good is signified by a flat, palm-down motion.

Emotions

Emotion is to be left off the court! Throwing a racket, hitting an erratic shot after play has stopped, and verbal outbursts should not be tolerated. An easy way to deal with opponents who behave in such an unacceptable manner is to refuse to play them. Life is too short to accept that sort of behavior in an environment that is supposed to be fun. Other unacceptable responses include making excuses for losing while not acknowledging the good play of an

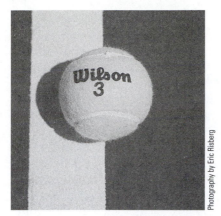

Photography by Eric Risberg

Photo 11.3 Ball on the line—"in."

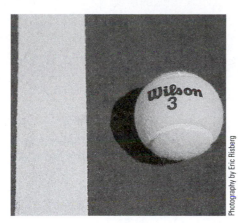

Photography by Eric Risberg

Photo 11.4 Ball near the line—"out."

opponent, and not keeping score accurately.

"In" and "Out"

Perhaps the most misunderstood part of etiquette is related to rules interpretation of when a ball is called "in" or "out" on a line call. The rule and the etiquette application are simple: A ball that touches any part of a court boundary line is "in" (Photo 11.3), and any time a ball is wholly out by not touching any part of a boundary line, the call is "out" (Photo 11.4).

The problem arises when players don't see the ball and start guessing. There is no excuse for guessing; that call is specific! If a player does not see a ball as "out," the ball must be considered playable, and it is communicated as good by continued play. There never is a guess on a line call in tennis: The ball is good unless it is seen to be out.

When it is unknown if a ball is in or out on the last play of a rally or on a serve, there is one exception to the call: If a player does not see the ball, that player can request that the other player make the call. If the opposing player was unsighted, or doesn't wish to make the call, the call reverts to the original player, who then must accept the ball as being in bounds.

Viewing a Match

Besides playing a tennis match and acknowledging etiquette, viewing a tennis match requires certain behavior, as a spectator has the obligation to observe a match with respect for the players. No communication should take place between player and spectator, including the often asked question, "What's the score?" The spectator should be quiet, watch the play, and applaud a good point. Spectator disruptions are not approved at major tennis tournament matches (such as the U.S. Open, professional tour matches, and collegiate competition).

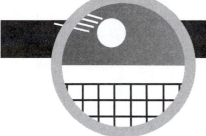

Points to Remember

Behavior on a Tennis Court

1. You must wear appropriate tennis shoes on a tennis court.

2. *Foot/racket pickup* and *ball-bounce pickup* are tennis skills related to picking up a ball off the court.

3. Wait until play has ceased on surrounding courts before walking onto your assigned tennis court.

4. "Ball please" and "thank you" are appropriate terms to request that a ball be returned from a court and to acknowledge the return.

5. A ball that is "in" play is acknowledged by continued play.

6. A ball that is "out" is acknowledged by stating "Out," or by pointing your index finger *up*.

7. A ball is always called in on any line call unless it is observed to be out.

8. If *unsighted,* it is appropriate to ask for an opponent to make a line call. If the opponent is *unsighted*, the ball must be ruled "in."

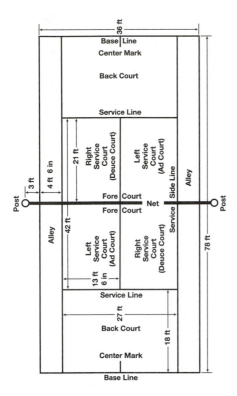

Figure 11.1 Court dimensions.

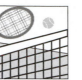

Interpreting Tennis Rules

Key terms include **baseline**, **center mark**, **backcourt**, **forecourt**, right **service court** (deuce), left **service court** (ad), **service line**, and the **alley**. (see Figure 11.1.) The singles court size is 27' × 78' and the expanded doubles court size is 36' × 78'. The net is 3'6" high at the net supports and 3' high at the center. The net height at the center is of particular importance, because a lower or higher height impacts the rally between two players.

The center net height is measured by placing one racket vertically at the center strap position and the other racket horizontally on top of the butt of the first racket's handle. Because most rackets today are oversized, the second string of the horizontal racket should be even with the top of the net for the net to be at the correct height (Photo 11.5).

Pre-play Choices

At the beginning of a match, significant choices to be made are choice of serve and side of court. A decision on choice of service and side of court to begin play is made by spinning the racket or flipping a coin. To spin a racket, place the top of the racket head on the court. The opposing player calls either "up" or "down" to signify the position of the butt end of the racket when it falls to the court. The winner of the spin chooses, or requests the opponent to choose, the right to be the server or receiver. The player who doesn't have first choice then selects the end of the court to begin play. The choices may be reversed, with the winner of the spin choosing, or requesting the opponent to choose, the end to begin play, followed by the non-selecting player's choice of service or receiving serve.

This scenario might clarify the choices available: Player A wins the spin and states, "I will serve." Player B then states, "I will take the north side." A second scenario consists of Player A winning the spin and stating, "Your choice." Player B then states, "I will receive," followed by Player A's rejoinder, "I will take the north side." The point is that the first player has the option of choosing service, receipt of serve, or end of the court, or of passing those choices to the opponent.

Order of Serve

In both singles and doubles play, the *order of serve* is a simple alternation of serves. A player must serve through a full game, then exchange service with the opponent at the conclusion of that game. In doubles, the situation is the same except that teams alternate serving following each game. If Team 1 serves the first game, Team 2 will serve game two, and the rotation will continue. Player A of Team 1 serves the first game, Player A of Team 2 serves the second game, Player B of Team 1 serves the third game, and Player B of Team 2 serves the fourth game. The sequence repeats throughout the set, with Player A of Team 1 serving in game five, etc.

Changing Sides of the Court

Changing sides of the court has a significant effect on performance when playing outdoors. Without changing the side of court, one player always faces the sun or wind during play, giving the opponent an advantage. Rotation to different sides of the court occurs when the total number of games played is an odd number.

If Player A (or Team 1) serves from the north side of a court in game one, sides will be exchanged for game two. Player B (or Team 2)

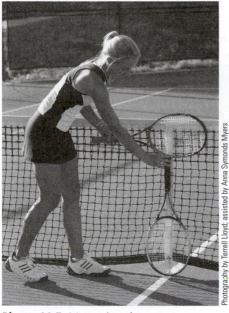

Photo 11.5 Measuring the net.

Photography by Terrell Lloyd; assisted by Anna Symonds Myers

Table 11.1 Point Scoring

Point Number	Equivalent Term
First point	15
Second point	30
Third point	40
Fourth point	game (must win by two points)
No points	love
Tie score	deuce
After a tie at 4 points each—server leads	advantage in (AD IN)
After a tie at 4 points each—receiver leads	advantage out (AD OUT)

then serves from the north side of the court, followed by Player A (or Team 1) serving game three from the south end of the court. At the conclusion of game three, the players (or teams) again change sides of the court, with Player B (or Team 2) serving from the south side of the court in game four.

The sequence continues with players (or teams) exchanging sides of the court at the conclusion of the fifth, seventh, ninth, and eleventh, etc. total games played. At the end of a set, the players or teams change sides only if the total games are an odd number (such as 6–3 for a total of nine games). In singles, the rotation of server is continuous throughout play of a set. In doubles, the same principle applies with the rotation of each team in order of service.

Doubles play has rules to control the *location of players while serving and receiving*. As with singles, once the serving rotation is determined for a team, as described, the rotation is permanent until a new set begins. The same is true for a team receiving the serve. One player always must receive from the right service court, and one player always must receive from the left service court. As with serving, the receiving order may be changed only at the start of a new set.

Scoring

When viewed systematically, scoring is simple to understand. A tennis match is played in a sequence of points, games, sets, and match. It takes 4 points to win a **game** (provided that the margin for victory is 2 points). A player must win six games to win a **set**, with a winning margin of two games.

One exception to the rule is that if each player wins six games, a tie-breaker is played to determine the winner, and the final score always will be 7-6—a margin of only one game for the victory. In most situations, the winner of the **match** is the winner of two of three sets (professional players on the men's tour play three of five sets in some tournaments).

Each point won by a player is assigned a term, as given in Table 11.1. Scores to complete a set are one of the following: 6–0, 6–1, 6–2, 6–3, 6–4, 7–5, or 7–6. If a set score reaches 5–5 in terms of games won, two more games must be played. If one player wins both games, the final score is 7–5. If the players split games, the score will be 6–6, and a tie-breaker will be played. Examples of a match score are 6–2, 7–5, or 6–3, 1–6, 6–4. The winning player's scores are always identified first in a match; consequently, the 1–6 score of the second set of the second

Table 11.2 Tie-Breaker Server Rotation

Singles				Doubles			
Player Number	Service Court to Serve To	Number of Points		Team No.	Player No.	Service Court to Serve To	Number of Points
1	Deuce Service Court	1		1	A	Deuce Service Court	1
2	Ad Service Court	1		2	A	Ad Service Court	1
2	Deuce Service Court	1		2	A	Deuce Service Court	1
1	Ad Service Court	1		1	B	Ad Service Court	1
1	Deuce Service Court	1		1	B	Deuce Service Court	1
2	Ad Service Court	1		2	B	Ad Service Court	1
change sides of court				change sides of court			
2	Deuce Service Court	1		2	B	Deuce Service Court	1
1	Ad Service Court	1		1	A	Ad Service Court	1
1	Deuce Service Court	1		1	A	Deuce Service Court	1
etc.				etc.			

match example indicates that the winner of the match lost the second set by a 6-to-1 game score.

Tie-Breakers

A *tie-breaker* is played only when a set is tied 6–6. There are several forms of tie-breakers, including what are called 7-, 9-, and 12-point tie-breakers. The 12-point tie-breaker is the most popular. The winner of the tie-breaker is the first player to win 7 points with a winning margin of 2 points. If the score in a tie-breaker reaches 6–6 in number of points scored, the players must continue the game until one player has a winning margin of 2 points (8–6, 9–7, 10–8, etc.). A 5–5 point score can still produce a winner at 7 points if one player wins the next 2 points.

The server for the first point of a tie-breaker is designated by the continued rotation of serve per the normal rotation. The first server serves only 1 point—from the **deuce service court**. The second server then begins the serve from the **ad service court**. This server serves one point from the ad service court, then one point from the deuce service court.

In singles, the service order now reverts to the first server, who begins service for 1 point from the ad service court, then moves to the deuce service court for the second point. The players exchange ends of court after a total of 6 points are played, with a continuation of the rotation.

In doubles play rotation, movement is the same as in singles except that four players are involved instead of two. Player A of Team 1 serves point number 1 to the deuce service court. Player A of Team 2 serves 2 points—one from the ad service court, followed by one from the deuce service court. Player B of Team 1 then serves points 1 and 2 from the respective ad and deuce service courts, and the rotation continues to Player B of Team 2, and so on. The tie-breaker singles and doubles rotations are presented in Table 11.2.

Numerous additional scoring possibilities include 8-game pro sets used in college matches, and 10-point tie breakers used in lieu of third sets. "No-Ad" scoring tends to be popular, as it speeds up play. No-ad scoring sequence is specific to a 3–3 point tie with the winner of the next point as the winner of a game.

The Ball in Play

Every game begins with a service to the right service court. The service point, both in a regular game situation and in a tie-breaker, allows a maximum of two opportunities to hit a legal serve. The one exception is a let, a serve that is hit in all ways legally except that the ball touches the net on its path to the service court. A let permits the server to repeat the serve, and any number of lets may be played in succession.

Once the ball is in play, a player must hit it over the net so it lands in the opponent's court. During a rally, players may hit the ball on the bounce or during flight (return of serve follows the bounce of the ball in the service court). A point is lost when

1. A ball bounces twice before being returned,
2. A ball lands out of the court boundaries on the fly,
3. A ball hits the net and does not go over the net, or
4. Two serves (excluding a let) in a row do not fall into the appropriate service court.

A serve that does not strike the appropriate service court is called a **fault**. Servers also fault by swinging and missing a service toss or by stepping on the baseline during the serve. Touching the service line on a serve is called a **foot fault**. Many players have the habit of touching the baseline in this manner, and legally that is not accepted. If a player strikes the ball, then comes down on the baseline, the serve is legal. When the foot touches the line while the racket is in contact with the ball, or prior to hitting the ball, the serve is lost. In "friendly" play, foot faults usually are ignored because they are difficult to see. But the server has a responsibility to avoid the illegal foot position.

Rule Infractions

Tennis has numerous rule infractions and interpretations. Some of them are as follows.*

1. Hitting a volley prior to the ball crossing the net is a loss of point except when a ball crosses the net and the wind blows or backspin carries the ball back across the net.
2. A ball that strikes the player or the player's clothing carries a loss of point.
3. Throwing a racket at the ball carries the penalty of loss of the point.
4. If the ball strikes the net (excluding the serve) and continues on into the opponent's court, the ball is still in play.
5. If a doubles player hits the partner with the ball, the team loses the point.
6. A receiver of a serve must be ready for service or the serve must be repeated.
7. An opposing player may not hinder an opponent by distracting the opponent; however, partners on a doubles team are allowed to talk to each other when the ball is directed to their side of the court.
8. A player hit by a ball prior to the ball striking the court loses that point even if the ball is going to land out of bounds.
9. After the conclusion of a tie-breaker, the first server of the next set is the player who did not serve first in the previously played set.

The beginning tennis player should treat the rules with respect and take them seriously so the game will be enjoyable.

---

* A review of USTA's *The Code: The Player's Guide for Unofficiated Matches* is found in Appendix A, by permission of the United States Tennis Association, Publications Department, 70 West Red Oak Lane, White Plains, NY 10604.

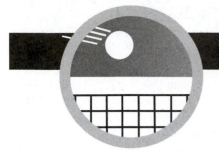

Points to Remember

Interpreting Tennis Rules

1. On the spin of the racket, the winner has the choices of electing to serve or receive, side of court, or to pass the choice to the opponent.

2. The order of service is a simple alternation of serves after each game is played.

3. Players change sides of the court on uneven total number of games.

4. A serve that doesn't strike the appropriate court is called a *fault*.

5. A set score is the first to six games with a winning margin of two games.

6. A score of 6–6 requires a 12-point tie-breaker.

7. A tie-breaker is played to 7 points with a winning margin of 2 points.

Checkpoints ✔✔

1. A ball that strikes the line of the court during play is considered
   a. a replay.
   b. out.
   c. in.
   d. none of the above.

2. Sides of the tennis court are changed by players after
   a. every third game.
   b. every odd total number of games accumulated by both players.
   c. every other game played.
   d. a player has an odd total number of games played.

3. Typically, an official legal score of a match is
   a. 6-3, 3-6, 6-5.
   b. 7-6, 3-6, 6-3.
   c. 5-6, 7-6, 7-5.
   d. 7-5, 5-7, 7-1.

4. Which of the following is not a legal score?
   a. Deuce
   b. Advantage In (Ad In)
   c. 15–love
   d. 45–15

5. A let is a
   a. serve that is hit legally but touches the net before falling into the opponent's service court.
   b. replay of a point when a call is considered in doubt.
   c. term used to say "take two."
   d. fault.

6. Hitting a volley shot while the ball is on the opponent's side of the court is considered
   a. loss of point.
   b. fair play.
   c. a replay.
   d. a mistake.

7. A tie-breaker is played
   a. when the game score is tied 5–5.
   b. when the game score is tied 6–6.
   c. any time there is a tie score in a game.
   d. until a player is ahead by 2 points.

8. It is poor etiquette to
   a. talk on the court.
   b. not wear appropriate tennis clothing.
   c. throw a tennis racket in anger.
   d. all of the above.

Answers to Checkpoints can be found on page 147.

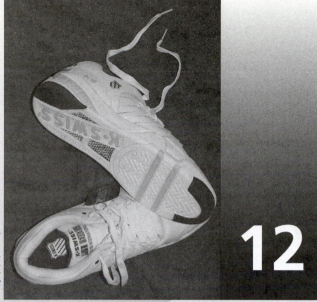

Photography by J.E. Bryant

12

Tennis Courts, Equipment Design, Tournament Competition, and Resources

At the beginning of the new millennium, tennis underwent a modest renewal in participation. Sales of balls—a barometer of a sport's health—were up 4.8 percent within the tennis market ("All in Favor," *Tennis*, December/January 2000, p. 18). This growth included all ages, the most dramatic of which is that 95 percent of newcomers to tennis were under 35 years of age and 54 percent were female ("All in Favor," p. 18).

As your tennis participation expands, your skills and knowledge base will also improve and contribute to your continual development. This chapter covers how a court is designed, which tennis racket to select, how to get involved in tennis competition, and what additional resources are available.

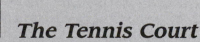

The Tennis Court

Tennis court surfaces are of five categories. *Grass courts* are traditional but have outlived their usefulness. Wimbledon is the only major professional tournament still played on a grass court. For normal play, the upkeep and expense involved in maintaining the surface is nearly prohibitive. Few grass courts are found in the United States, and they are nearly extinct worldwide.

Soft courts are popular throughout much of the world and east of the Mississippi River in the United States. The typical soft court is a *clay court*. Its surface provides a high bounce and a slow ball that encourage long baseline rallies. The term "clay court" is descriptive of what used to be the surface composition of a claylike material and coarse sand. A number of other claylike surfaces include shale and synthetic composites that result in play like clay.

Today a "clay court" is composed of a two-layer base of crushed limestone with ⅛" of brick dust, or a one-layer base of crushed and firmly packed stone material called "fast-dry." The clay surface poses a maintenance problem when reasonable play conditions are desired, because it requires watering and rolling, but

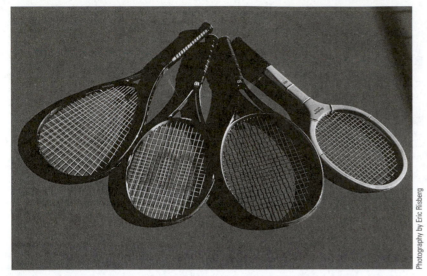

Photography by Eric Risberg

Photo 12.1 Comparison of wood and composite wide-body rackets.

the more recent surfaces are easier to maintain.

All-weather or *hard court* surfaces are extremely popular in the United States. This is the surface with which most developing players are familiar. The surface may be composed of asphalt or cement topping, which contributes to ease of maintenance and cleaning. Courts with this surface are usually public, and they are easily recognized because they give a uniform, fast-bouncing action to the ball.

The *synthetic surface* is another type of hard surface that many players have used on their college campuses. The synthetic court surface usually is composed of a series of granulated rubber particles pulled together with an epoxy resin sprayed with a polyurethane coating and laid on a porous foundation. The court is designed to play like a naturally made court, but it is free of maintenance and cleaning problems. The synthetic court is called the Mercury Grassphalts Court.

Another court surface, called a *carpet,* is used for indoor tournaments on the professional tennis tour. The carpet is laid over whatever existing surface is available, and that combination produces a fast court that encourages a serve-volley game.

Hard and synthetic courts are smoothed or roughened depending on the amount of play and rally circumstances expected in a given geographical area. High-altitude locations tend to have a roughened surface to provide more opportunity for baseline play. Courts in low altitudes tend to have a smoother surface, as the density of the air allows for more rally situations.

Tennis Equipment

Tennis Rackets

At one time, tennis rackets were made of various woods including ash or beech and combinations of perhaps sycamore, obeche, or mahogany. The wood racket was hand-crafted, and the number of wood laminations indicated the quality of the racket. Wood rackets now are obsolete, replaced by modern technology's new materials (Photo 12.1).

Following wood rackets, tennis rackets were designed with metal and aluminum materials, but these, too, are all but obsolete. The tennis racket of the 21st century is made of materials such as polyurethane, carbon, Kevlar, fiberglass, graphite, and titanium. These materials provide more power with control, reduced racket vibration and shock, and a lighter racket for quicker reaction for stroke readiness.

Wide-body and Extra-long Rackets Wide-body rackets emerged as a popular racket just a few years ago. They provided maximum power with increased control and bent less at contact, giving the ball more energy.

The most recent technology has produced a racket that is more elongated than any previous racket. These long-body or *extra-long rackets* provide increased power, enhanced spin, and far more leverage when

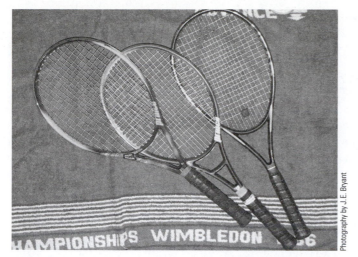

Photography by J.E. Bryant

Photo 12.2 Assorted long-body tennis rackets.

striking the ball. They enable a player to reach balls hit wide to them, and because they are so light, they provide the player with the ability to move the racket more quickly in order to set up to hit a shot. The extra-long rackets (also called *stretch rackets*) typically are made of titanium and graphite, and they range from 27.5" to 29" in length (Photo 12.2).

Trends in Rackets and Heads

Head size for today's rackets ranges generally from 85 square inches to 125 square inches. The larger the head size, the more power can be generated; the smaller the head size, the more control. A mixture of power and control for head size should be between 100 square inches and 105 square inches. The heavier a racket, the more power, but today's rackets are all basically light. Weight ranges from 8–9.8 ounces for super light-weight rackets, to 9.9–10.8 ounces for light rackets, to 10.9 ounces and above for heavy rackets. A light racket provides greater maneuverability, while concealing shock and vibration. A heavier racket provides additional power.

A typical example of a racket prototype designed for beginning and intermediate players might be 27.5 square inches in length, 105 square inches racket face, a weight of 9.25 oz., of titanium mesh (titanium woven with graphite). This prototype, as reflected in extra-long rackets, is now the most widely sold type of racket.

Mid-size rackets with less length and racket-face surface have emerged as the racket most used by highly skilled players. This level of play does not require enhanced racket technology. Rackets have changed in size over the last 15 years, ranging from a regular size to a mid-size to an oversize racket. The Prince racket was the first over-size racket, and now all companies are manufacturing oversize rackets. Shapes of racket heads range from pear-shaped to round to oblong.

Characteristics of Rackets A stiff racket bends less on impact and offers less control and more power than a flexible racket. A flexible racket will provide more control but less power. Often, 27-inch-length rackets have more flexibility, and wide-body and extra-long rackets tend to be more stiff, thus providing more power. A rule of thumb is that a racket length of 28.5" to 29" is a stiff, powerful racket; a length of 27.5" to 28" provides a combination of power and control; and a 27" length is designed more for control.

Typically the beginner needs a flexible racket with some stiffness to provide some power or zip to the ball. As skill is developed, more stiffness or more flexibility becomes a personal choice.

A flexible racket also tends to reduce vibration and shock, which decreases the potential for developing *tennis elbow* (tendonitis). **Vibration** describes a lingering back and forth motion of the racket frame and strings after the ball has been hit. Torque from vibration then is transferred to the elbow. *Shock* describes the contact of string to ball, and when a ball is hit off-center, a subsequent twisting action also generates a torque action that is transferred to the elbow. In both

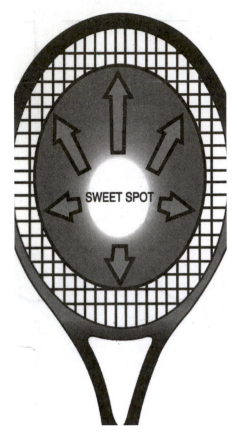

Figure 12.1 Sweet spot.

cases, the transfer of shock or vibration to the elbow contributes to tendonitis of the elbow.

Other characteristics of a tennis racket, *power, control, feel, maneuverability, comfort, and stability*, are used in tennis publications and racket advertisements. Rackets also are characterized as head-light, balanced, and head-heavy. And they are light, semi-light, and medium in weight.

Sweet Spot   The ideal area for contact with the ball is called a **sweet spot** (Figure 12.1). It can be located below center, above center, elongated, or wide across center. Most sweet spots are found at center and above center, but they do vary. Sweet spots basically allow for a shot that is hit not quite on center to still rebound effectively.

The larger the oversize racket, the larger is the sweet spot—and the more chance for success. A stiffer racket stretches the sweet spot, and lowering the string tension increases a sweet spot's effectiveness ("Sweet Talk About the Sweet Spot," by S. Chirls, *Tennis,* June 1992, p. 77).

Grips   Racket grips are measured from 4⅛" to 4⅞". The most widely used grips range from 4¼" to 4⅝". Grips are composed of several types of material, but a cushioned grip with a tacky feel that is perforated or embossed is recommended.

A grip should feel comfortable. Grip size is determined by a simple measure. Grasp the racket handle with an eastern forehand grip. When looking at your grip, there should be a space between the fingertips of your hand and the palm. If you can place the index finger of your non-racket hand snugly between the fingertips and the palm of the racket hand and the grip feels comfortable, you have a fit.

Strings   Rackets are purchased unstrung if they are of reasonable quality. Tennis rackets are strung with gut or synthetic nylon strings.

Gut is a high-quality string that has limited durability but great feel. Synthetic strings are designed to replace the feel of gut with a far more durable quality. A number of synthetic strings provide a combination of durability and holding their tension. The four types are: monofilaments, multifilaments, aramids, and polyester.

1. *Monofilaments* are composed of a single, solid-core string, encased in a thin outer cover. They are the most popular string for a tennis racket, as they hold their tension and provide both durability and playability.

2. *Multifilaments* consist of thousands of individual fibers woven together to form one piece of a string. They provide more power but are not as durable as monofilaments.

3. *Aramids* are made of Kevlar or Technora, and they are the most durable, but they do not provide much in the way of feel or power ("String Fever," by D. Dusek, *Tennis,* April 1999, pp. 64–65).

4. *Polyester* strings have become more popular, as they tend not to break (D. Dusek, *Tennis,* April 2000, pp. 53–54).

Racket strings also are defined by size, and when a racket is strung (Photo 12.3), the string is measured in amount of tension applied to the racket. String size is measured in gauge. A thinner string (e.g., 16-gauge) increases power and spin, while a thicker 15 gauge is more durable but generates less power and spin. String tension is measured in pounds of tension. The higher the tension, the more control, but with less durability (string breaks). Lower tension enhances power.

Costs   Tennis rackets are expensive. So are strings. A high-performance tennis racket usually retails for $135–$300, and to string a racket is an added $18–$35. Based on the

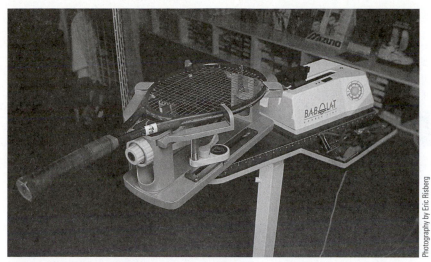

Photo 12.3 Tennis stringer.

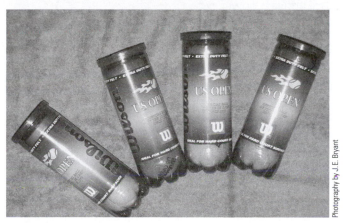

Photo 12.4 Tennis balls.

above discussion regarding rackets, you have enough information to make a decision on what kind of racket to purchase. As a beginner you don't need a $300 racket. You don't even need a $135 racket. But you do need a racket that has as many qualities as possible that meet your needs, and one that is within your price range.

Look for a racket with flexibility (control) and a good feel. Check to determine what features the racket has that seem similar to what has been described. And check out the cost. Most sporting goods stores have "loaners," which allow you to try out the rackets. Take advantage

of the loaner opportunity and play with different rackets. Pick one in your price range that meets your needs.

When you buy a racket, chances are that you also will have to have it strung, so apply the above information to the choice of a string. You are best off with a monofilament string, but select one in your price range when you start out as a player.

Tennis Balls

A can of tennis balls ranges from $2 to $4 and lasts only 2 or 3 hours of play (if play is continuous and skillful). Discount stores and major sporting goods dealers often run specials for less than $2, but the player should be aware that many types of tennis balls are sold at that price.

Regular-duty balls, with a tighter, thinner cover, tend to not "fluff" up. Extra-duty balls are thicker and more durable. Beginners and, for that matter, most times players, should look for premium and championship balls. An additional checkpoint for tennis balls is to be aware of "feel." For true bounce and longevity, balls should be a name brand. In the United States three companies—Wilson, Penn, and Dunlop—make approved tennis balls. Each company sells several types. Dunlop balls play "hard," Penn balls are "softer," and Wilson balls are in between.

Tennis balls are made of molded rubber. Two cups are cemented together, covered with a wool material, and inflated with compressed air. They then are placed in a pressure-sealed container, ready to be used when you are ready to play with a new group of three tennis balls. Pressurized balls don't last as long as hard-core rubber tennis balls, but they are easier on elbows and they play with a true bounce (Photo 12.4).

The hard-core ball has a greater life expectancy but begins to bounce too high after extensive play. There is a difference in ball bounce when playing at sea-level and playing at 5,000 feet. Tennis balls designed for sea-level play bounce much higher at altitude, so a high-altitude ball allows for a bounce adjustment and players who live at high altitudes should purchase only high-altitude balls.

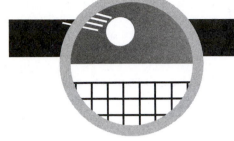

Points to Remember

Tennis Courts and Equipment

1. Tennis courts come in many surfaces, the most popular of which is either an all-weather court (hard court) or a synthetic hard court surface.

2. Extra-long tennis rackets are the most popular and effective racket available today. That is a stiff racket that allows the player more reach and more power.

3. Stiff rackets offer less control and more power whereas flexible rackets provide more control and less power.

4. Rackets are rated on qualities including control, maneuverability, vibration, shock, comfort, and feel.

5. The most durable, yet quality synthetic string designed for a tennis racket is a monofilament string.

6. Tennis strings are measured by their gauge size, and rackets are strung based on number of pounds of tension.

7. You can measure the fit of your tennis racket grip by placing your non-racket index finger in the space between the fingertips and the palm of your racket-hand grip.

Tennis Clothing

Selecting tennis shorts or skirt and a tennis top is up to the player. An investment of $10 for a pair of shorts and a tee-shirt to an expenditure in excess of $200 for designer tennis shorts and top is the range for purchase of clothing.

Tennis shoes (Photo 12.5) are a different matter expense-wise. They are never inexpensive. The tennis shoe is designed specifically for use on a tennis court and for the player's forward, backward, and lateral movement.

Tennis shoes are sized like regular shoes, and some tennis shoes also are measured in widths of wide or narrow. A tennis shoe must have a firm insole and a good arch support. The back portion of the shoe that rests against the Achilles tendon has to be soft and pliable, with an absorbent heel cushion. A tennis shoe also should have durability, be comfortable, and have good traction.

The toe of a tennis shoe is vulnerable to dragging and wearing out. Checking to determine how much abuse the toe of the shoe will take will help the player avoid a new purchase every 3 or 4 weeks. If the tennis shoe fits the player, if it provides good support, and if it won't wear out in a few weeks, it probably will cost $45 or more, but it is what a player ought to buy.

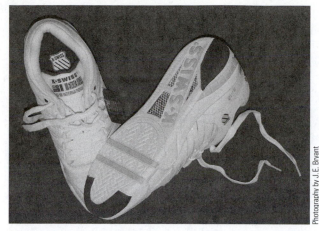

Photo 12.5 Tennis shoes.

Tennis socks are not all that expensive, but they have to be selected carefully. You want a sock that leaves a little room for your toes, moves moisture away from your skin to an outer layer of the cotton of the sock, and has a cushion for the soles of your feet. Look for a tennis sock that is made of cotton, has either a polyester fiber or a polyolefin fiber called Drylon to eliminate the excess sweat that contributes to blisters. Finally, to be fashionable, select either a low or below-the-calf-length sock that is white.

How to Get Started in Tennis Competition

A wide assortment of tennis tournaments takes place in the United States. Those that are of most interest to the beginning player are associated with recreation programs, college campus recreation programs, city tournaments, and club programs. There are tournaments for all types of players, from the novice who is just learning to hit a volley shot without ducking to a highly skilled player.

Tournaments usually are ladder tournaments, single-elimination or double-elimination tournaments, inter-club, tournaments, or social round-robin mixed doubles tournaments. Some are more competitive than others, and the player has to understand which are the more competitive and which are designed as social functions. With the proper perspective, all are fun to play.

Ladder tournaments are found in all situations, including most campus recreation programs. They allow players to play at their own level by challenging individuals of similar skill who are positioned higher on the ladder. Club competition is a highly competitive league-type of play in which records are kept and league standings are established. Rewards are given to the team finishing first and second in a league, with a team or teams advancing to another round of competitive play.

Many programs have single- and double-elimination tournaments with ratings, including novice, C, B, A, and open divisions. Most are sanctioned by the *United States Tennis Association* (USTA) and require membership in that organization to participate. Most USTA tournaments are identified by a rating scale, usually through the USTA National Tennis Rating Program. There also are age-division tournaments that have an open competition under 35 years of age, then age divisions, including 35 and over, 40 and over, 45 and over, 55 and over, 65 and over, and so on.

Most single- or double-elimination tournaments are played through a 3-day weekend, and a player may play five or six matches if the play continues all the way to the championship. The number of matches depends on the size of a draw for the tournament (a draw is the number of entrants).

The *USTA National Rating Program* has become popular for rating players, not only for tournament play but also for social play, to help players identify their level of skill so a match can be an equal competition. The rating scale is established from 1.0 through 7.0. The lower the rating classification, the closer to a beginner, and the higher the rating, the closer to a professional player. The classification of 3.0 to 5.0 seems to be the typical club player rating and probably is a major first goal for a developing player. The beginner usually starts at the 1.0 through the 2.5 level and progresses rapidly through the early classifications. The rating program provides a descriptive version of each classification, and many tennis teachers now are able to use the rating objectively and systematically. The great thing is that you can rate yourself based on how you compare your skills with the NTRP rating categories. Appendix B gives you a view of the National Tennis Rating Program categories.

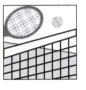

Tennis Resources

Numerous textbooks, periodicals, videos, and the Internet are available to help you to learn to play tennis and to continue to develop skills and knowledge associated with the game. Also, tennis associations have been formed to promote the game in community and tennis club environments.

The USTA is the most well known agency or organization with the goal of promoting tennis at every level of play and competition. To play in sanctioned USTA tournaments, membership in the USTA is required. The same group sponsors the National Tennis Rating Program. The USTA also publishes *Tennis* and *Tennis USTA*. Other publications produced by the USTA include general textbooks, material for group instruction and for teaching tennis, strategy material, program planning, tennis information, and rules/regulations.

Membership with the USTA is a small investment for the beginning player. The benefits for a serious player are excellent, and the organization really does function to promote tennis. The USTA membership address is: USTA/ Membership Department/ 70 West Red Oak Lane/ White Plains, NY 10604.

The USTA also has sectional offices and state organizations. The major role of these groups is to promote tennis. They also sponsor tennis tournaments. With a USTA membership, the member receives newsletters from sectional and state organizations. The local, state, and sectional organizations also rate players and carry on the work of the USTA.

Tennis publications and the Internet provide a plethora of instructional materials for the avid tennis player. Of the many tennis books on the market, five that serve as a nice supplement to *Game/Set/Match* are:

- *The Inner Game of Tennis Revised*, by W. Timothy Gallwey (New York: Random House, 1997, 122 pp.)

  A revised version of Gallwey's classic tennis book on mind, body connection, and relaxed concentration.

- *International Book of Tennis Drills*, by the U.S. Professional Tennis Registry (Chicago: Triumph Books, 1998, 289 pp.)

  An extensive series of tennis drills to enhance tennis skill development and strategy insight.

- *Sports Psychology Library: Tennis*, by Judy L. Van Raalte and Carrie Silver–Bernstein (Morgantown, WV: Fitness Information Technology, 1999, 135 pp.)

  Covers mental skills, building confidence, improving concentration, how to focus, how to play big matches, etc.

- *Tennis 2000–Strokes, Strategy, and Psychology*, by Vic Braden and Bill Burns (Boston: Little, Brown & Co., 1998, 284 pp.)

  Covers a biomechanical analysis of tennis fundamentals through photos and provides a complete analysis of tennis.

- *Tennis Injury Handbook: Professional Advice for Amateur Athletes,* by Allan M. Levy M.D. and Mark L. Feurst (New York: John Wiley & Sons, 1999, 185 pp.)

  Includes techniques for stretching, conditioning, rehabilitation, how to avoid court-side aches and pains, and how to recognize and heal injuries.

The Internet is a reference source that will continually change, but it is a fascinating option for finding information and instructional help regarding tennis. If you are interested in information associated with tennis results and stories, the assortment of major choices include:

CBS.Sportsline

CNN/SI

ESPN. Sportszone

Excite Sports

Foxsports.com

Nando-Tennis

MSNBC - Sports

USA Today. Tennis

If you are interested in Web sites with instructional analysis, general tennis information, and new ideas regarding tennis try:

- *Welcome to Tennis One* www.tennisone.com

  An excellent tennis instructional site.

- *The Tennis Serve* Center Court for Tennis on the Internet www.tennisserver. com

  A newsletter website that is a great source for just about any instructional or informational item that might be of interest.

- *Tennis Links—The Ultimate Website* www. tennislinks.com

  An excellent source of tennis links for equipment, tournaments, and general tennis information.

- *International Hall of Fame* www.tennisfame.org

  Official site for the Tennis Hall of Fame.

- *United States Tennis Association* www.usta.com

  Official site for the USTA office; includes extensive information regarding membership, the organization, and countless tennis-related information.

Television provides extensive coverage of major tennis events including the Australian Open, French Open, U.S. Open, and Wimbledon. In addition, smaller tournaments surface on television, along with an occasional collegiate tennis competition. These are instructional in the sense that, by watching skilled players, you can pick up new techniques, skills, and a feel for the game.

A final but important resource for a player who continues to develop after group instruction at the college/university level is a teaching professional. As an occasional review, or to have technique analyzed, a teaching professional is of value. The professional should be able to present the mechanics of stroke execution in an interesting and informative way, and should be able to analyze stroke mistakes.

Finding a teaching pro who is appropriate for you requires some effort. Look for teaching pros affiliated with tennis clubs who have credentials. What is their teaching background? Are they certified as a teaching professional? Do they come with good recommendations from former students?

Selecting of the proper resources is important and must be done with some insight. A player needs to keep up with changes in tennis, and to have enough knowledge to discuss tennis intelligently.

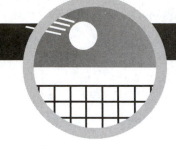

Points to Remember

Tennis Competition and Resources

1. Be sure to read and identify NTRP Rating Categories. Identify where you fit, and use that rating as a measure for improvement.

2. Once you have acquired a skill level at which you are comfortable with your play, seek out a tennis tournament that fits your skill level.

3. Countless tennis resources are available. Refer to the list of supplemental books and Web site addresses to explore the tennis Internet.

Checkpoints ✔✔

1. The tennis court surface used by most players is
   a. clay.
   b. grass.
   c. all-weather (hard court).
   d. synthetic.

2. A stiff racket has
   a. more control and less power than a flexible racket.
   b. more power and less control than a flexible racket.
   c. both more control and power than a flexible racket.
   d. both less control and power than a flexible racket.

3. A typical racket grip size ranges from
   a. $4\frac{1}{8}$ to $4\frac{5}{8}$ inches.
   b. $4\frac{3}{8}$ to $4\frac{7}{8}$ inches.
   c. $4\frac{1}{8}$ to $4\frac{7}{8}$ inches.
   d. $4\frac{1}{8}$ to $4\frac{3}{8}$ inches.

4. The sweet spot of a tennis racket can be found
   a. above center.
   b. in the center.
   c. wide across the center.
   d. all of the above.

5. Important characteristics to consider when buying tennis shoes include:
   a. Firm insole and good arch support.
   b. Absorbent heel cushion and a soft, pliable heel cup.
   c. Neither a nor b.
   d. Both a and b.

6. The most resilient, long-lasting, and inexpensive string used for a tennis racket is
   a. synthetic gut.
   b. gut.
   c. nylon.
   d. none of the above.

7. A player who is consistent when hitting medium placed shots, but not comfortable when trying for directionality, depth, or power is rated as
   a. a 2.5 player.
   b. a 3.0 player.
   c. a 3.5 player.
   d. a 4.0 player.

8. The USTA's major publication is
   a. *International Tennis Players*.
   b. *Tennis*.
   c. *Racquet*.
   d. *World Tennis*.

9. Other tennis resources besides magazines include:
   a. Nando—Tennis
   b. www.tennislinks.com
   c. Gallwey's *The Inner Game of Tennis*
   d. All of the above

10. An instructional source for tennis players following taking a class is
    a. a teaching professional.
    b. playing matches.
    c. neither a nor b.
    d. both a and b.

Answers to Checkpoints can be found on page 147.

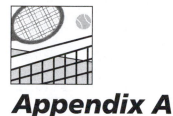

Appendix A

USTA's The Code: The Player's Guide for Unofficiated Matches

Preface

When your serve hits your partner stationed at the net, is it a let, fault, or loss of point? Likewise, what is the ruling when your serve, before touching the ground, hits an opponent who is standing back of the baseline. The answers to these questions are obvious to anyone who knows the fundamentals of tennis, but it is surprising the number of players who don't know these fundamentals. All players have a responsibility to be familiar with the basic rules and customs of tennis. Further, it can be distressing to your opponent when he makes a decision in accordance with a rule and you protest with the remark: "Well, I never heard of that rule before!" Ignorance of the rules constitutes a delinquency on the part of a player and often spoils an otherwise good match.

What is written here constitutes the essentials of The Code, a summary of procedures and unwritten rules which custom and tradition dictate all players should follow. No system of rules will cover every specific problem or situation that may arise. If players of good will follow the principles of The Code, they should always be able to reach an agreement, while at the same time making tennis more fun and a better game for all. The principles set forth in The Code shall apply in cases not specifically covered by The Rules of Tennis and USTA Regulations.

Before reading this you might well ask yourself: Since we have a book that contains all the rules of tennis, why do we need a code? Isn't it sufficient to know and understand all the rules? There are a number of things not specifically set forth in the rules that are covered by custom and tradition only. For example, if you have a doubt on a line call, your opponent gets the benefit of the doubt. Can you find that in the rules?

Further, custom dictates the standard procedures that players will use in reaching decisions. These are the reasons why we need a code.

—Col. Nick Powel

Note: This edition of The Code is an adaptation of the original, which was written by Colonel Nicholas E. Powel.

General Principles

1. Courtesy. Tennis is a game that requires cooperation and courtesy from all participants. Make tennis a fun game by praising your opponents' good shots and by not:
   - conducting loud postmortems after points;
   - complaining about shots like lobs and drop shots;
   - embarrassing a weak opponent by being overly gracious or condescending;
   - losing your temper, using vile language, throwing your racket, or slamming a ball in anger; or
   - sulking when you are losing.
2. Counting points played in good faith. All points played in good faith stand. For example, if after losing a point, a player discovers that the net was four inches too high, the point stands. If a point is played from the wrong court, there is no replay. If during a point, a player realizes that a mistake was made at the beginning (for example, service from the wrong court), he shall continue playing the point. Corrective action may be taken only after a point has been completed.

Reprinted Courtesy of the USTA

The Warm-up

3. Warm-up is not practice. A player should provide his opponent a five-minute warm-up (ten minutes if there are no ball persons). If a player refuses to warm-up his opponent, he forfeits his right to a warm-up. Some players confuse warm up and practice. A player should make a special effort to hit his shots directly to his opponent. (If partners want to warm each other up while their opponents are warming up, they may do so.)

4. Warm-up serves. Take all your warm-up serves before the first serve of the match. Courtesy dictates that you not practice your service return when your opponent practices his serve. If a player has completed his warm-up serves, he shall return warm-up serves directly to his opponent.

Making Calls

5. Player makes calls on his side of the net. A player calls all shots landing on, or aimed at, his side of the net.

6. Opponent gets benefit of doubt. When a match is played without officials, the players are responsible for making decisions, particularly for line calls. There is a subtle difference between player decisions and those of an on-court official. An official impartially resolves a problem involving a call, whereas a player is guided by the unwritten law that any doubt must be resolved in favor of his opponent. A player in attempting to be scrupulously honest on line calls frequently will find himself keeping a ball in play that might have been out or that he discovers too late was out. Even so, the game is much better played this way.

7. Ball touching any part of line is good. If any part of the ball touches the line, the ball is good. A ball 99% out is still 100% good.

8. Ball that cannot be called out is good. Any ball that cannot be called out is considered to have been good. A player may not claim a let on the basis that he did not see a ball. One of tennis' most infuriating moments occurs after a long hard rally when a player makes a clean placement and his opponent says: "I'm not sure if it was good or out. Let's play a let." Remember, it is each player's responsibility to call all balls landing on, or aimed at, his side of the net. If a ball can't be called out with certainty, it is good. When you say your opponent's shot was really out but you offer to replay the point to give him a break, you are deluding yourself because you must have had some doubt.

9. Calls when looking across a line or when far away. The call of a player looking down a line is much more likely to be accurate than that of a player looking across a line. When you are looking across a line, don't call a ball out unless you can clearly see part of the court between where the ball hit and the line. It is difficult for a player who stands on one baseline to question a call on a ball that landed near the other baseline.

10. Treat all points the same regardless of their importance. All points in a match should be treated the same. There is no justification for considering a match point differently than the first point.

11. Requesting opponent's help. When an opponent's opinion is requested and he gives a positive opinion, it must be accepted. If neither player has an opinion, the ball is considered good. Aid from an opponent is available only on a call that ends a point.

12. Out calls corrected. If a player mistakenly calls a ball "out" and then realizes it was good, the point shall be replayed if he returned the ball within the proper court. Nonetheless, if the player's return of the ball results in a "weak sitter," the player should give his opponent the point. If the player failed to make the return, his opponent wins the point. If the mistake was made on the second serve, the server is entitled to two serves.

13. Player calls his own shots out. With the exception of the first serve, a player should call against himself any ball he clearly sees out regardless of whether he is requested to do so by his opponent. The prime objective in making calls is accuracy. All players should cooperate to attain this objective.

14. Partners' disagreement on calls. If a player and his partner disagree about whether their opponents' ball was out, they shall call it good. It is more important to give your opponents the benefit of the doubt than to avoid possibly hurting your partner's feelings by not overruling. The tactful way to achieve the desired result is to tell your partner quietly that he has made a mistake and then let him overrule himself. If a call is changed from out to good, the point is replayed only if the out ball was put back in play.

15. Audible or visible calls. No matter how obvious it is to a player that his opponent's ball is out, the opponent is entitled to a prompt audible or visible out call.

16. Opponent's calls questioned. When a player genuinely doubts his opponent's call, the player may ask: "Are you sure of your call?" If the opponent reaffirms that the ball was out, his call shall be accepted. If the opponent acknowledges that he is uncertain, he loses the point. There shall be no further delay or discussion.

17. Spectators never to make calls. A player shall not enlist the aid of a spectator in making a call. No spectator has a part in the match.

18. Prompt calls eliminate two chance option. A player shall make all calls promptly after the ball has hit the court. A call shall be made either before the player's return shot has gone out of play or before the opponent has had the opportunity to play the return shot.

Prompt calls will quickly eliminate the "two chances to win the point" option that some players practice. To illustrate, a player is advancing to the net for an easy put away when he sees a ball from an adjoining court rolling toward him. He continues his advance and hits the shot, only to have his supposed easy put away fly over the baseline. The player then claims a let. The claim is not valid because he forfeited his right to call a let by choosing instead to play the ball. He took his chance to win or lose, and he is not entitled to a second chance.

19. Lets called when balls roll on the court. When a ball from an adjacent court enters the playing area, any player shall call a let as soon as he becomes aware of the ball. The player loses the right to call a let if he unreasonably delays in making the call.

20. Touches, hitting ball before it crosses net, invasion of opponent's court, double hits, and double bounces. A player shall promptly acknowledge if:

- a ball touches him;

- he touches the net;

- he touches his opponent's court;

- he hits a ball before it crosses the net;
- he deliberately carries or double hits the ball; or
- the ball bounces more than once in his court.

21. Balls hit through the net or into the ground. A player shall make the ruling on a ball that his opponent hits through the net and on a ball that his opponent hits into the ground before it goes over the net.

22. Calling balls on clay courts. If any part of the ball mark touches the line on a clay court, the ball shall be called good. If you can see only part of the mark on the court, this means that the missing part is on the line or tape. A player should take a careful second look at any point-ending placement that is close to a line on a clay court. Occasionally a ball will strike the tape, jump, and then leave a full mark behind the line. The player should listen for the sound of the ball striking the tape and look for a clean spot on the tape near the mark. If these conditions exist, the player should give the point to his opponent.

Serving

23. Server's request for third ball. When a server requests three balls, the receiver shall comply when the third ball is readily available. Distant balls shall be retrieved at the end of a game.

24. Foot Faults. A player may warn his opponent that the opponent has committed a flagrant foot fault. If the foot faulting continues, the player may attempt to locate an official. If no official is available, the player may call flagrant foot faults. Compliance with the foot fault rule is very much a function of a player's personal honor system. The plea that he should not be penalized because he only just touched the line and did not rush the net is not acceptable. Habitual foot faulting, whether intentional or careless, is just as surely cheating as is making a deliberate bad line call.

25. Service calls in doubles. In doubles the receiver's partner should call the service line, and the receiver should call the sideline and the center service line. Nonetheless, either partner may call a ball that he clearly sees.

26. Service calls by serving team. Neither the server nor his partner shall make a fault call on the first service even if they think it is out because the receiver may be giving the server the benefit of the doubt. But the server and his partner shall call out any second serve that either of them clearly sees out.

27. Service let calls. Any player may call a service let. The call shall be made before the return of serve goes out of play or is hit by the server or his partner. If the serve is an apparent or near ace, any let shall be called promptly.

28. Obvious faults. A player shall not put into play or hit over the net an obvious fault. To do so constitutes rudeness and may even be a form of gamesmanship. On the other hand, if a player believes that he cannot call a serve a fault and gives his opponent the benefit of a close call, the server is not entitled to replay the point.

29. Receiver readiness. The receiver shall play to the reasonable pace of the server. The receiver should make no effort to return a serve when he is not ready. If a player attempts to return a serve (even if it is a "quick" serve), then he (or his team) is presumed to be ready.

30. Delays during service. When the server's second service motion is interrupted by a ball coming onto the court, he is entitled to two serves. When there is a delay between the first and second serves:

- the server gets one serve if he was the cause of the delay;
- the server gets two serves if the delay was caused by the receiver or if there was outside interference.

The time it takes to clear a ball that comes onto the court between the first and second serves is not considered sufficient time to warrant the server receiving two serves unless this time is so prolonged as to constitute an interruption. The receiver is the judge of whether the delay is sufficiently prolonged to justify giving the server two serves.

Scoring

31. Server announces score. The server shall announce the game score before the first point of the game and the point score before each subsequent point of the game.

32. Disputes. Disputes over the score shall be resolved by using one of the following methods, which are listed in the order of preference:

- count all points and games agreed upon by the players and replay only the disputed points or games;
- play from a score mutually agreeable to all players;
- spin a racket or toss a coin.

Hindrance Issues

33. Talking during a point. A player shall not talk while the ball is moving toward his opponent's side of the court. If the player's talking interferes with his opponent's ability to play the ball, the player loses the point. Consider the situation where a player hits a weak lob and loudly yells at his partner to get back. If the shout is loud enough to distract his opponent, then the opponent may claim the point based on a deliberate hindrance. If the opponent chooses to hit the lob and misses it, the opponent loses the point because he did not make a timely claim of hindrance.

34. Feinting with the body. A player may feint with his body while the ball is in play. He may change position at any time, including while the server is tossing the ball. Any movement or sound that is made solely to distract an opponent, including but not limited to waving the arms or racket or stamping the feet, is not allowed.

35. Lets due to hindrance. A let is not automatically granted because of hindrance. A let is authorized only if the player could have made the shot had he not been hindered. A let is also not authorized for a hindrance caused by something within a player's control. For example, a request for a let because the player tripped over his own hat should be denied.

36. Grunting. A player should avoid grunting and making other loud noises. Grunting and other loud noises may bother not only opponents but also players on adjacent courts. In an extreme case, an opponent or a player on an adjacent court may seek the assistance of the referee or a roving official. The referee or official may treat grunting and the making of loud noises as a hindrance. Depending upon the circumstance, this could result in a let or loss of point.

37. Injury caused by a player. When a player accidentally injures his opponent, the opponent suffers the

consequences. Consider the situation where the server's racket accidentally strikes the receiver and incapacitates him. The receiver is unable to resume play within the time limit. Even though the server caused the injury, the server wins the match by retirement.

On the other hand, when a player deliberately injures his opponent and affects the opponent's ability to play, then the opponent wins the match by default. Hitting a ball or throwing a racket in anger is considered a deliberate act.

When to Contact an Official

38. Withdrawing from a match or tournament. A player shall not enter a tournament and then withdraw when he discovers that tough opponents have also entered. A player may withdraw from a match or tournament only because of injury, illness, personal emergency, or another bona fide reason. If a player cannot play a match, he shall notify the referee at once so that his opponent may be saved a trip. A player who withdraws from a tournament is not entitled to the return of his entry fee unless he withdrew before the draw was made.

39. Stalling. The following actions constitute stalling :
    - warming up for more than the allotted time;
    - playing at about one-third a player's normal pace;
    - taking more than the allotted 90 seconds on the odd-game changeover;
    - taking a rest at the end of a set that contains an even number of games;
    - taking more than the authorized ten minutes during an authorized rest period between sets;
    - starting a discussion or argument in order for a player to catch his breath;
    - clearing a missed first service that doesn't need to be cleared; and
    - bouncing the ball ten times before each serve.

    Contact an official if you encounter a problem with stalling. It is subject to penalty under the Point Penalty System.

40. Requesting an official. While normally a player may not leave the playing area, he may visit the referee or seek a roving official to request assistance. Some reasons for visiting the referee include:
    - stalling;
    - chronic flagrant foot faults;
    - a medical time-out
    - a scoring dispute; and
    - a pattern of bad calls.

    A player may refuse to play until an official responds.

Ball Issues

41. Retrieving stray balls. Each player is responsible for removing stray balls and other objects from his end of the court. A player shall not go behind an adjacent court to retrieve a ball, nor shall he ask for return of a ball from players on an adjacent court until their point is over. When a player returns a ball that comes from an adjacent court, he shall wait until their point is over and then return it directly to one of the players, preferably the server.

42. Catching a ball. Unless you have made a local ground rule, if you catch a ball before it bounces, you lose the point regardless of where you are standing.

43. New balls for a third set. When a tournament specifies new balls for a third set, new balls shall be used unless all the players agree otherwise.

Miscellaneous

44. Clothing and equipment malfunction. If clothing or equipment other than a racket becomes unusable through circumstances outside the control of the player, play may be suspended for a reasonable period. The player may leave the court after the point is over to correct the problem. If a racket or string is broken, the player may leave the court to get a replacement, but he is subject to code violations under the Point Penalty System.

45. Placement of towels. Place towels on the ground outside the net post or at the back fence. Clothing and towels should never be placed on the net.

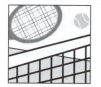

Appendix B

NTRP Rating Categories

Guidelines

The rating categories are generalizations about skill levels. You may find that you actually play above or below the category which best describes your skill level, depending on your competitive ability. The category you choose is not meant to be permanent, but may be adjusted as your skills change or as your match play demonstrates the need for reclassification.

To place yourself:

A. Begin with 1.0. Read all categories carefully and then decide which one best describes your present ability level.

B. Be certain that you qualify on all points of all preceding categories as well as those in the classification you choose.

C. When rating yourself assume you are playing against a player of the same gender and the same ability.

D. If you are undecided between 2 NTRP levels, you should place yourself in the higher level of play.

E. **Ultimately your true NTRP rating is based upon your match results**, so use match play history against players who have an established NTRP rating as a major indicator of your true NTRP level.

NTRP 1.0

This player is just starting to play tennis.

NTRP 1.5

This player has limited experience and is still working primarily on getting the ball over the net, has some knowledge of scoring but is not familiar with the basic positions and procedures for singles and doubles play.

NTRP 2.0

This player may have had some lessons but needs on-court experience; has obvious stroke weaknesses but is beginning to feel comfortable with singles and doubles play.

Forehand: Incomplete swing; lacks directional intent

Backhand: Avoids backhands; erratic contact; grip problems; incomplete swing

Serve/Return of Serve: Incomplete service motion; double faults common; toss is inconsistent; return of serve erratic

Volley: Reluctant to play net; avoids backhand; lacks footwork

Playing Style: Familiar with basic positions for singles and doubles play; frequently out of postion

NTRP 2.5

This player has more dependable strokes and is learning to judge where the ball is going; has weak coverage or is often caught out of position, but is starting to keep the ball in play with other players of the same ability.

Forehand: Form developing; prepared for moderately paced shots

Backhand: Grip and preparation problems; often chooses to hit forehand instead of backhand

Serve/Return of Serve: Attempting a full swing; can get the ball in play at slow pace; inconsistent toss; can return slow paced serves

Volley: Uncomfortable at net especially on the backhand side; frequently uses forehand racket face on backhand volleys

Special Shots: Can lob intentionally but with little control; can make contact on overheads

Playing Style: Can sustain a short rally of slow pace; weak court coverage; usually remains in the initial doubles position

NTRP 3.0

This player can place shots with moderate success, can sustain a rally of slow pace but is not comfortable with all strokes; lacks control when trying for power.

Forehand: Fairly consistent with some directional intent; lacks depth control

Backhand: Frequently prepared; starting to hit with fair consistency on moderate shots

Serve/Return of Serve: Developing rhythm; little consistency when trying for power; second serve is often considerably slower than first serve; can return serve with fair consistency

Volley: Consistent forehand volley; inconsistent backhand volley, has trouble with low and wide shots

Special Shots: Can lob consistently on moderate shots

Playing Style: Consistent on medium-paced shots; most common doubles formation is still one-up, one-back;

approaches net when play dictates but weak in execution

NTRP 3.5

This player has achieved improved stroke dependability and direction on shots within reach, including forehand and backhand volleys, but still lacks depth and variety; seldom double faults and occasionally forces errors on the serve.

Forehand: Good consistency and variety on moderate shots; good directional control; developing spin

Backhand: Hitting with directional control on moderate shots; has difficulty on high or hard shots; returns difficult shots defensively

Serve/Return of Serve: Starting to serve with consistency and some power, developing spin; can return serve consistently with directional contol on moderate shots

Volley: More aggressive net play; some ability to cover side shots; uses proper footwork; can direct forehand volleys; controls backhand volley but with little offense; difficulty in putting volleys away

Special Shots: Consistent overhead shots within reach; developing approach shots, drop shots, and half volleys; can place the return of most second serves

Playing Style: Consistency on moderate shots with directional control; improved court coverage; starting to look for the opportunity to come to the net; developing teamwork in doubles

NTRP 4.0

This player has dependable strokes on both forehand and backhand sides; has the ability to use a variety of shots including lobs, overheads, approach shots and volleys; can place the first serve and force some errors; is seldom out of position in a doubles game

Forehand: Dependable; hits with depth and control on moderate shots; may try to hit too good a placement on a difficult shot

Backhand: Player can direct the ball with consistency and depth on moderate shots; developing spin

Serve/Return of Serve: Places both first and second serves; frequent power on first serve; uses spin; dependable return of serve; can return with depth in singles and mix returns in doubles

Volley: Depth and control on forehand volley; can direct backhand volleys but usually lacks depth; developing wide and low volleys on both sides of the body

Special Shots: Can put away easy overheads; can poach in doubles; follows

aggressive shots to the net; beginning to finish point off; can hit to opponent's weaknesses; able to lob defensively on setups; dependable return of serve

Playing Style: Dependable ground strokes with directional control and depth demonstrated on moderate shots; not yet playing good percentage tennis; teamwork in doubles is evident; rallies may still be lost due to impatience

NTRP 4.5

This player has begun to master the use of power and spins; has sound footwork; can control depth of shots and is able to move opponent up and back; can hit first serves with power and accuracy and place the second serve; is able to rush net with some success on serve in singles as well as doubles

Forehand: Very dependable; uses speed and spin effectively; controls depth well; tends to overhit on difficult shots; offensive on moderate shots

Backhand: Can control direction and depth but may break down under pressure; can hit power on moderate shots

Serve/Return of Serve: Aggressive serving with limited double faults; uses power and spin; developing offense; on second serve frequently hits with good depth and placement; frequently hits aggressive service returns; can take pace off with moderate success in doubles

Volley: Can handle a mixed sequence of volleys; good footwork; has depth and directional control on backhand; developing touch; most common error is still overhitting

Special Shots: Approach shots hit with good depth and control; can consistently hit volleys and overheads to end the point; frequently hits aggressive service returns

Playing Style: More intentional variety in game; is hitting with more pace; covers up weaknesses well; beginning to vary game plan according to opponent; aggressive net play is common in doubles; good anticipation; beginning to handle pace

NTRP 5.0

Player has good shot anticipation; frequently has an outstanding shot or exceptional consistency around which a game may be structured; can regularly hit winners or force errors off of short balls; can successfully execute lobs, drop shots, half volleys and overhead smashes; has good depth and spin on most second serves

Forehand: Strong shot with control, depth, and spin; uses forehand to set up

offensive situations; has developed a good touch; consistent on passing shots

Backhand: Can use backhand as an aggressive shot with good consistency; has good direction and depth on most shots; varies spin

Serve/Return of Serve: Serve is placed effectively with the intent of hitting to a weakness or developing an offensive situation; has a variety of serves to rely on; good depth, spin, and placement on most second serves to force weak return or set up next shot; can mix aggressive and off-paced service returns with control depth, and spin

Volley: Can hit most volleys with depth, pace, and direction; plays difficult volleys with depth; given opportunity, volley is often hit for a winner

Special Shots: Approach shots and passing shots are hit with pace and a high degree of effectiveness; can lob offensively; overhead can be hit from any position; hits mid-court volley with consistency; can mix aggressive and off-paced service returns

Playing Style: Frequently has an outstanding shot or attribute around which his game is built; can vary game plan according to opponent; this player is "match wise," plays percentage tennis, and "beats himself" less than the 4.5 player; solid teamwork in doubles is evident; game breaks down mentally and physically more often than the 5.5 player

NTRP 5.5

This player can execute all strokes offensively and defensively; can hit dependable shots under pressure; is able to analyze opponents' styles and can employ patterns of play to assure the greatest possibility of winning points; can hit winners or force errors with both first and second serves. Returns of serve can be an offensive weapon.

NTRP 6.0

This player has mastered all the above skills, has developed power and/or consistency as a major weapon; and can vary strategies and styles of play in a competitive situation. This player typically has had intensive training for national competition at junior or college levels.

NTRP 6.5

This player has has mastered all of the above skills and is an experienced tournament competitor who regularly travels for competition and whose income may be partially derived from prize winnings.

NTRP 7.0

This is a world class player.

Answer Key to Checkpoints

Chapter 1
1-a, 2-c, 3-d, 4-a, 5-a, 6-b, 7-d, 8-c

Chapter 2
1-b, 2-a, 3-c, 4-b, 5-d, 6-d, 7-a, 8-b, 9-c, 10-d

Chapter 3
1-d, 2-a, 3-a, 4-c, 5-d, 6-a, 7-a, 8-d

Chapter 4
1-d, 2-a, 3-a, 4-d, 5-c, 6-b, 7-c, 8-a, 9-d, 10-c

Chapter 5
1-c, 2-c, 3-a, 4-d, 5-a, 6-a, 7-c, 8-b

Chapter 6
1-b, 2-d, 3-c, 4-b, 5-a, 6-c, 7-d, 8-b

Chapter 7
1-a, 2-a, 3-b, 4-b, 5-c, 6-d, 7-a, 8-b

Chapter 8
1-a, 2-a, 3-c, 4-d, 5-c, 6-d, 7-c, 8-c

Chapter 9
Refer to the various skill drills in the chapter and your skill level

Chapter 10
1-d, 2-Refer to the discussion on stretching pp. 110–111, 3-Refer to the discussion on stretching pp. 110–111, 4-a, 5-c, 6-a, 7-a, 8-c

Chapter 11
1-c, 2-b, 3-b, 4-d, 5-a, 6-a, 7-b, 8-d

Chapter 12
1-c, 2-b, 3-a, 4-d, 5-d, 6-c, 7-b, 8-b, 9-d, 10-c

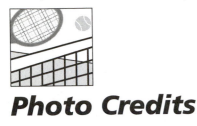

Photo Credits

Cover Image Ken Reid/Getty Images

Chapter One
p. 1 Photography by Eric Risberg; p. 2 Photography by Eric Risberg; p. 3 Photography by Eric Risberg; p. 4 Photography by Terrell Lloyd; assisted by Anna Symonds Myers; p. 5 Photography by Terrell Lloyd; assisted by Anna Symonds Myers; p. 6 Photography by Terrell Lloyd; assisted by Greg Harris and Tim May; p. 7 Photography by Terrell Lloyd; assisted by Anna Symonds Myers; p. 9 Photography by Eric Risberg

Chapter Two
p. 13 Photography by Terrell Lloyd; assisted by Anna Symonds Myers; p. 14 Photography by Terrell Lloyd; assisted by Anna Symonds Myers; p. 15 (top left) Photography by Terrell Lloyd; assisted by Anna Symonds Myers; (top center, top right, center left) Photography by Eric Risberg; p. 16 Photography by Terrell Lloyd; assisted by Anna Symonds Myers; (inset) Photo by Eric Risberg; p. 18 (top left, bottom left, bottom right) Photography by Terrell Lloyd; assisted by Anna Symonds Myers; (inset) Photo by Eric Risberg; (top right) Photography by Eric Risberg; p. 19 (left) Photography by Eric Risberg; (center, right) Photography by Terrell Lloyd; assisted by Anna Symonds Myers; p. 20 Photography by Terrell Lloyd; assisted by Anna Symonds Myers; (inset) Photo by Eric Risberg; p. 22 Photography by Terrell Lloyd; assisted by Anna Symonds Myers; (inset) Photo by Eric Risberg; p. 24 Photography by Terrell Lloyd; assisted by Anna Symonds Myers; p. 25 Photography by Eric Risberg; p. 26 Photography by Eric Risberg; p. 27 Photography by Terrell Lloyd; assisted by Anna Symonds Myers; (insets) Photos by Eric Risberg; p. 28 Photography by Terrell Lloyd; assisted by Anna Symonds Myers; p. 29 Photography by Terrell Lloyd; assisted by Anna Symonds Myers

Chapter Three
p. 33 Photography by Terrell Lloyd; assisted by Anna Symonds Myers; p. 34 Photography by Terrell Lloyd; assisted by Anna Symonds Myers; (inset) Photo by Eric Risberg; p. 35 Photography by Terrell Lloyd; assisted by Anna Symonds Myers; p. 36 Photography by Terrell Lloyd; assisted by Anna Symonds Myers; p. 38 Photography by Terrell Lloyd; assisted by Anna Symonds Myers; p. 39 Photography by Terrell Lloyd; assisted by Anna Symonds Myers; p. 40 Photography by Terrell Lloyd; assisted by Anna Symonds Myers

Chapter Four
p. 43 (top) Photography by Terrell Lloyd; assisted by Anna Symonds Myers; (bottom) Photography by Terrell Lloyd; assisted by Anna Symonds Myers; (inset) Photo by Eric Risberg; p. 44 Photography by Terrell Lloyd; assisted by Anna Symonds Myers; p. 45 Photography by Eric Risberg; p. 46 Photography by Terrell Lloyd; assisted by Anna Symonds Myers; p. 48 Photography by Terrell Lloyd; assisted by Anna Symonds Myers; p. 49 Photography by Terrell Lloyd; assisted by Anna Symonds Myers; p. 50 Photography by Terrell Lloyd; assisted by Anna Symonds Myers; p. 52 Photography by Terrell Lloyd; assisted by Anna Symonds Myers; p. 53 Photography by Terrell Lloyd; assisted by Anna Symonds Myers; (inset) Photo by Eric Risberg

Chapter Five
p. 57 Photography by Terrell Lloyd; assisted by Anna Symonds Myers; p. 58 Photography by Terrell Lloyd; assisted by Anna Symonds Myers; (inset) Photo by Eric Risberg; p. 59 Photography by Terrell Lloyd; assisted by Anna Symonds Myers; (inset) Photo by Eric Risberg; p. 62 Photography by Terrell Lloyd; assisted by Anna Symonds Myers; (insets) Photos by Eric Risberg; p. 63 Photography by Terrell Lloyd; assisted by Anna Symonds Myers; (inset) Photo by Eric Risberg; p. 64 (top) Photography by Terrell Lloyd; assisted by Anna Symonds Myers; (inset) Photo by Eric Risberg; (center) Photography by Terrell Lloyd; assisted by Anna Symonds Myers; p. 65 Photography by Terrell Lloyd; assisted by Anna Symonds Myers

Chapter Six
p. 67 Photography by Terrell Lloyd; assisted by Anna Symonds Myers

Chapter Seven
p. 75 Photography by Terrell Lloyd; assisted by Anna Symonds Myers; p. 77 Photography by Terrell Lloyd; assisted by Anna Symonds Myers; p. 79 Photography by Terrell Lloyd; assisted by Anna Symonds Myers; p. 82 Photography by Terrell Lloyd; assisted by Anna Symonds Myers; p. 84 Photography by Terrell Lloyd; assisted by Anna Symonds Myers

Chapter Eight
p. 87 Photography by Terrell Lloyd; assisted by Anna Symonds Myers; p. 88 Photography by Terrell Lloyd; assisted by Anna Symonds Myers; p. 89 Photography by Terrell Lloyd; assisted by Anna Symonds Myers; p. 90 Photography by Terrell Lloyd; assisted by Anna Symonds Myers; p. 91 Photography by Terrell Lloyd; assisted by Anna Symonds Myers

Chapter Nine
p. 97 Photography by Terrell Lloyd; assisted by Anna Symonds Myers; p. 100 Photography by Terrell Lloyd; assisted by Anna Symonds Myers; p. 101 Photography by Terrell Lloyd; assisted by Anna Symonds Myers; p. 102 Photography by Terrell Lloyd; assisted by Anna Symonds Myers; p. 103 Photography by Terrell Lloyd; assisted by Anna Symonds Myers; p. 104 Photography by Terrell Lloyd; assisted by Anna Symonds Myers; p. 105 Photography by Terrell Lloyd; assisted by Anna Symonds Myers; p. 106 Photography by Terrell Lloyd; assisted by Anna Symonds Myers; p. 107 Photography by Terrell Lloyd; assisted by Anna Symonds Myers

Chapter Ten
p. 109 Photography by Terrell Lloyd; assisted by Anna Symonds Myers; p. 110 Photography by Terrell Lloyd; assisted by Anna Symonds Myers; p. 111 Photography by Terrell Lloyd; assisted by Anna Symonds Myers; p. 112 Photography by Terrell Lloyd; assisted by Anna Symonds Myers

Chapter Eleven
p. 123 Photography by Terrell Lloyd; assisted by Anna Symonds Myers; p. 124 Photography by Eric Risberg; p. 125 Photography by Eric Risberg; p. 127 Photography by Terrell Lloyd; assisted by Anna Symonds Myers

Chapter Twelve
p. 131 Photography by J. E. Bryant; p. 132 Photography by Eric Risberg; p. 133 Photography by J. E. Bryant; p. 135 (top) Photography by Eric Risberg; (center) Photography by J. E. Bryant; p. 137 Photography by J. E. Bryant

Glossary of Terms

Ad: Advantage of one point to the server or receiver in a tie game.

Ad service court: The left service court.

Ad in: Advantage to the server.

Ad out: Advantage to the receiver.

Aerial game: Overhead smashes and defensive and offensive lobs as part of the total tennis game.

Aerobic: Literally, "with oxygen."

Alley: Space on the court between singles and doubles sidelines.

American twist service: Serve that has a reverse side spin applied to the ball.

Anaerobic: The release of energy without using oxygen.

Anxiety: Mental pressure that reduces physical performance.

Approach shot: A groundstroke hit inside the baseline toward the net.

Australian doubles: A two-player alignment in doubles that places the net player in a position perpendicular from server to the net.

Backcourt: Area of the tennis court defined between service court back line and baseline. Extends beyond baseline for purpose of understanding the concept of standing in that area to return a groundstroke.

Backhand: Balls hit on the non-racket side of the body.

Ballistic movement: Physically moving the body to prepare for a match.

Baseline: The end of the court, located 39 feet from the net.

Center mark: The division line on the baseline that separates the right side from the left side of the court.

Center strap: The strap that anchors the middle of the net to the court at a 3-foot height.

Chop: An exaggerated slice stroke.

Closed face: Position of the racket face as it is turned down toward the court.

Complex overhead: Includes a scissors kick as the player jumps to hit the ball.

Control: The measure of how effectively the racket permits the player to place the ball on various shots.

Conventional doubles: Two players in a doubles match who are positioned as one up (at net), one back (at baseline).

Close in: Move in on the net following an approach shot, an overhead, or a volley.

Cross-court: Hitting the ball at an angle across the width of the court with the net as the central boundary.

Defensive lob: A ball hit to give the defending player a chance to recover from an opponent's offensive shot.

Deuce: A tie score in games at 40–40 or beyond.

Deuce service court: The right side service court.

Dink shot: A sidespin drop shot hit at an angle from the net to the other side of the court.

Division line theory of play: The division of the court between the opponent's position and the other player's position that provides an equal distance to reach a forehand or a backhand shot.

Double fault: Serving two illegal serves during one service point.

Down the line: A shot hit down a sideline in a direct line from the player.

Drive: A ball hit with force.

Drop shot: A ball hit from a groundstroke position that barely clears the net and dies on the opponent's side of the court.

Drop volley: Same shot as drop shot but from a position of hitting the ball before it bounces on the court.

Dump shot: A push action that guides the ball to an open area beyond the opponent's side of the court.

Eye-hand coordination: The coordination between visual observation and hand reaction.

Etiquette: Rules of behavior on a tennis court.

Fault: An illegally hit serve.

Feel: The general kinesthetic sense of how a racket feels in the hand of the player.

Flat serve: A serve hit with little spin and with a basically flat trajectory.

Flexible racket: A tennis racket that has more control and less power.

Focus: The ability to concentrate on seeing and hitting the ball while eliminating outside influences.

Foot fault: An illegal serve due to foot touching baseline before or at contact with the ball.

Forecourt: Area of the tennis court between the net and the service court line.

Forehand: Balls hit on the racket side of the body.

Game: First player to win 4 points with a winning margin of 2 points.

Groundstroke: The act of hitting a ball following the bounce of the ball on the court.

Gut: Type of racket string.

Half-volley: A ball hit immediately following the bounce on the court.

Homebase: The position assumed by a player who prefers to play from the baseline and rally.

Ladder tournaments: A challenge form of tournament often played in club tennis.

Let: A point played over because of interference or a serve replayed because of an otherwise legal serve touching the net.

Lob: A ball hit up over the net player, driving that player back away from the net.

Longbody: An extra long racket.

Loop: A groundstroke backswing action that is defined by a high backswing position to contact with the ball.

Love: A zero score.

Match: The best two of three sets in most play situations.

Moonball: A lofted topspin shot intended to change the pace of a rally; halfway between a lob and a groundstroke.

Net play: Generally, offensive play near the net with volley shots and approach shots characteristic of the shots hit.

No Man's Land: The area on the court between the service court line and baseline where a player should never set up to begin a rally.

Non-racket shoulder: The shoulder of the arm on which the racket is not grasped (right-hand player's non-racket shoulder is the left shoulder).

Non-racket side of the body: The same description as for non-racket shoulder, but refers to the whole side of the body (right-handed player's left side of the body).

Offensive lob: A lofted shot hit deep to opponent's baseline with topspin ball action used to chase opponent away from the net.

Open racquet face: Position of racket face as it is turned up to the sky.

Orthodox overhead: An overhead that requires no foot position exchange.

Overhead stroke: An offensive throwing action stroke similar to a serve in motion but delivered at the net, back to the baseline.

Pace: A ball hit with the same consistency, usually with some degree of velocity.

Percentage tennis: A philosophical strategy based on forcing the opponent to make the error rather than one's hitting all winning shots.

Playability: A subjective measure of how the racket responds in general during play.

Power: Also described as a "sweet spot," the measure of the "power zone" of the racket.

Punching action: Hitting the ball with little backswing or follow-through.

Racket face: The strings of the racket as they face the oncoming ball during a stroke sequence.

Racket head: The total racket area including the string and the material around the face.

Racket shoulder: The shoulder of the arm with which the player grasps the racket.

Racket side of the body: Same description as for the racket shoulder but including the whole side of the body.

Rally: Sustained play of a point, usually associated with hitting only groundstrokes from the baseline area; never refers to hitting a ball on the fly, as in a volley.

Ready position: The foundation position a player assumes prior to initiating a stroke in tennis. Term is usually used as a ready position for a groundstroke or a volley shot.

Return of serve: The act of hitting a ball back off a serve.

Service court: Area of court for placement of a serve.

Service court line: The line that is the base of the service courts and that is parallel to the net and baseline.

Set: Represents the winning of six games with a margin of two games, or winning by a score of 7–5 or 7–6.

Sidespin: Spin action imparted on a tennis ball so the ball will land on the court and kick away from the person hitting the ball; ball is hit on the backside portion to give the sidespin effect.

Slice: A ball hit with sidespin.

Social doubles: Tennis played in a friendly atmosphere with a player alignment usually of one up, one back.

Stability: Ability of a racket to resist the twisting motion when the ball is hit off center.

Static stretching: A stretch that places the muscle in a fixed position.

Stiff racket: A tennis racket that has less control and more power.

Strategy: The planning of an attack when competing against another player or a doubles team.

Stretch racket: An extra long racket or longbody racket.

Stretch warm-up: Static stretching of muscle groups to prepare for a match.

Sweet spot: Surface area of the racket face that provides a functional rebound area as the ball strikes the racket at contact.

Swinging action: A groundstroke movement that represents the motor pattern of swinging as in a baseball bat swing.

Throwing action: A serving or overhead motion used to strike a tennis ball that represents a throwing pattern as in throwing a baseball.

Timing: The coordinated effort of hitting a ball at the right synchronized point.

Topspin: A ball hit with an overspin rotation action.

Topspin serve: A serve that has a forward or overspin rotation applied to the ball; end result is a high-bouncing, quick rebound from the tennis court.

Underspin: A ball hit with backspin rotation; the ball will have a tendency to float and slow down when striking the tennis court.

Volley: A shot hit before ball bounces on the court.

Vibration: The measure of how well a racket absorbs vibration at contact with the ball.

Warm-up: Physically preparing for a tennis match by working the muscles and stretching.

Warm down: Cooling off the body in a sequential, logical order upon finishing a tennis match.

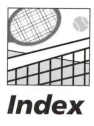

Index